The Castrated Woman

Naomi Miller Stokes

The CASTRATED WOMAN

What Your Doctor Won't Tell You About Hysterectomy

FRANKLIN WATTS   1986   NEW YORK/TORONTO

Epigraph from "In Celebration of My Uterus"
in *Love Poems* by Anne Sexton.
Copyright 1967, 1968, 1969 by Anne Sexton.
Reprinted by permission of Houghton Mifflin Company.

Library of Congress Cataloging-in-Publication Data

Stokes, Naomi Miller.
The castrated woman.

Bibliography: p.
Includes index.
1. Hysterectomy.   2. Hysterectomy—Psychological
aspects.   3. Hysterectomy—Patients—Interviews
I.   Title.
RG391.S65 1986   362.1'981453   86-1522
ISBN 0-531-15003-8

Contents

Acknowledgments

Just as no person lives in a vacuum, so no book is created in a space empty of others. My space, while I was working on this book, was brightened and enriched by these very important people without whom the book would not be:

First of all, the many women who shared their experiences with me, in the hope that knowledge will become prevention.

Michael Larsen and Elizabeth Pomada, my wonderfully *alive* agents, whose aspirations for their clients are just as lofty as the San Francisco street on which they live and work.

Elizabeth R. Hock, senior editor at Franklin Watts, Inc., who guided me around the worst shoals of emotionalism, and who is the best thing that can happen to an author—an excellent editor.

Don James, patron saint of Pacific Northwest writers, who first told me, "You've got a book. Write it."

Victor Gregory, M.D., prominent west coast psychiatrist, who, when I said, "But I'm not a doctor. Will anyone listen?," replied the best reply of all, "You're a woman. And that's even better."

Edwin Weinstein, M.D., friend, fellow author and Devil's Advocate.

Marlene Howard, whose ear and shoulder were always available, especially when they were most needed, and whose enthusiasm ignited many a gray day.

Linda Lay Shuler, my fellow author, who waded through first drafts and offered numerous helpful and pertinent suggestions.

Lola Janes, mistress of the limerick, whose place at Seaside was the scene of much contemplation as well as actual writing.

Melinda Stokes Richards, who, being literate, brilliant and twenty-five years younger, provided her mother with many invaluable insights.

To my husband, Joe;
My four children,
David, Melinda, Matthew, and Megan;
And my three small granddaughters,
Heather, Meagan, and newborn Sarah,
All of whom have taught me
the various dimensions of love.

The Castrated Woman

In Celebration of My Uterus

They wanted to cut you out
But they will not . . .
They said you were sick unto dying
But they were wrong.

You are singing like a school girl.

Anne Sexton

Foreword

As I write this foreword (November, 1985) to Naomi Miller Stokes's crucially important book, the assault of "modern medicine" on the sexual organs of women has reached record levels.

The masked man (and woman!) armed with a scalpel took out—according to the latest annual statistics—an all-time high of 800,000 uteruses in 1985. And, not satisfied with the decades-old bloodshed due to the discredited, but by no means abandoned, radical mastectomy, the doctor has added to his breast repertoire the "prophylactic" (subcutaneous) mastectomy. Furthermore, his slaughter during childbirth has yielded, in addition to an undiminished harvest of episiotomies, a 30 percent-plus Cesarean section rate.

Yet, in accord with Newton's Law—which applies to human affairs as well as to physics—the counterattack against this surgical juggernaut is mounting. In this war for human survival, Naomi Miller Stokes's publication provides a powerful weapon. She claims her book is about *love*. I would add—it is about *life*.

This book is must-reading for the following audiences:

—every woman threatened with a hysterectomy
—every woman who has had a hysterectomy
—every man whose woman falls into the above two categories

1

—every parent of a woman in those two categories
—every young girl about to begin menses who wants a lyrical, yet rational, description of menstruation
—every attorney, especially trial lawyers specializing in malpractice and personal injury, faced with women who have suffered grave damage without ever having received the information necessary to make a decision on the basis of informed consent.

Armed with the information presented by Mrs. Stokes, women will increasingly be able to resist the doctor who threatens them with the "Big C" should they fail to accept his advice. Only when patients become more fearful of the scalpel than of the cancer will the body count begin to drop.

The Castrated Woman appears just at the right time, together with the emergence of the new consumer health movement in the United States. Citizens throughout the country are now organizing to fight the major cause of illness today—iatrogenic (Greek for "doctor-produced") disease.

The Castrated Woman will evoke a profound response in every citizen dedicated to the eradication of injustice, especially the deadly injustice of hysterectomy.

Robert S. Mendelsohn, M.D.
Author, *MALePRACTICE:*
How Doctors Manipulate Women

Preface

This book is about hysterectomy in America today. It is neither a medical textbook nor a political treatise; it is an exploration of what happened to me following a complete hysterectomy, a statement that grew out of my need to understand and explain the mysterious changes I underwent, and an account of what happened to other women following the surgery. In short, it offers the good news, the bad news, the discoveries—some of which border on revelation, viable alternatives, and hope.

For decades the medical profession has assured women that removal of the uterus and ovaries is a benign surgery, that it will have no adverse effects on their bodies or on their sexuality; that, on the contrary, sex will be better. For some women, this is true. But countless women have found it to be untrue and, in the finding, have been labeled "a little strange"— seriously in need of psychological attention.

Loss of sexual desire and enjoyment following hysterectomy strikes untold thousands of women. It is a physical problem, not a mental or an emotional one; if, however, it is allowed to go unresolved, it can become either one or both.

Sexual dysfunction is just one sequela of a crippling surgery that is being performed with increasing frequency. Other tragic aftereffects include a sharp rise in the incidence of atherosclerotic heart disease and crippling and painful osteoporosis as well as severe depression that has led, in some cases, to suicide attempts.

In my own search for the truth about hysterectomy, I began by talking to women I knew. They talked to their friends, who called and talked to me. I wrote to friends around the country who, in turn, had women in their locales write or call me. The network spread. I put aside my discomfort about asking intimate questions.

What I found was an almost unbelievable conspiracy of silence. I discovered that I was by no means alone but that only those who have been there—who have walked out of the operating rooms of this country minus their "women's organs"— know and speak the truth about hysterectomy.

During my research, I suffered a near-fatal heart attack and underwent bypass surgery. I was diagnosed as having developed atherosclerotic heart disease, now known as a frequent result of loss of ovarian and uterine function.

The more I heard and studied, the angrier I grew. I sold my business and devoted my time to discovering what is going on with women and hysterectomy in this country today. For the most part, it is not good.

During my seven years of research I interviewed 500 women from all walks of life and from all over the United States regarding their experiences with the aftermath of hysterectomy. The body of testimony, the anecdotal evidence, is astounding.

Of these 500 women, 51 did not know whether they still had their ovaries; 12 considered sex better after the surgery; 38 considered their operations absolutely necessary; 234 had the surgery for birth control reasons, although they said their doctors put "other reasons" on the medical forms; 477 did not care as much for sex after the surgery; 399 lost sexual appetite entirely; 473 were under 44 years of age.

Of the 477 who suffered from some degree of libido loss, all felt that had they been told beforehand that sexual dysfunction *could* occur, they and their mates would have been far more able to deal with it. The biggest problem was being told the surgery could in no way cause such problems when they suffered from these problems every night in their bedrooms. Too often the legacy of hysterectomy is a troubled marriage, leading, in many cases, to divorce, usually within two to five years of the surgery. Sometimes the woman's personality changes to such a degree she no longer has any feeling for her mate. Sometimes the man leaves. These are men who have been otherwise devoted partners but who can no longer endure either a robot-like sexual relationship or a downright sexless one.

Upon rare occasions I encountered women who were happy with their hysterectomies. The records show that these women were divided into three distinct categories. The first were women who had suffered nearly unbearable pain during certain phases of their menstrual cycles; for them, surgery provided relief. The second were women who felt extremely protective of their doctors, exhibiting, along with some anger, feelings of "my doctor is God and he is not to be questioned"; these women also evidenced a personalization and extreme possessiveness regarding their surgeries, referring to them continually as "*my* hysterectomy." The third group were women who, since girlhood, had detested their menstrual periods, considering them crippling disabilities that prevented them from participating in sports with their male peers.

In writing this book I have been helped immeasurably by many concerned medical people, both men and women. Hysterectomy is a highly controversial subject as well as a highly emotional one. Happily, the doors of awareness are opening. Only a few years ago virtually no one in the medical profession would admit that many women suffer loss of libido after hysterectomy. Now it is known to be a fact, but the reasons for it are energetically disputed.

The Castrated Woman began as an inward journey, a search for something of inestimable value that had been lost. It grew with the realization that I was not alone and that sexual dysfunction is only one of the disorders hysterectomy may leave in its wake. During my search I discovered that there is hope for the castrated woman. I also discovered that there are alternate therapies that in many cases can spare a woman a hysterectomy. When women understand *before* the fact of surgery what hysterectomy can do to their systems, they will demand these alternate therapies.

This book is our contribution—mine, the women and men I interviewed, my medical sources—to any woman contemplating hysterectomy, to those women who have already undergone the surgery, and to those who love these women. Most of all, it is for my daughters who, I hope, will never wear the "smiling scar."

Naomi Miller Stokes
Portland, Oregon
1986

Prologue

"Do you want your uterus?" the doctor asked as he ripped off his examining gloves and flung them into the stainless steel sink.

"Do I want my uterus?" I was too astonished to do more than repeat his question from the discomfort of the classic pelvic examination position on Dr. Jones's table. "Of course I want my uterus."

"Why?" He was half-turned from me as he scrubbed his hands carefully, one finger at a time.

I paused to consider the question. Why *did* I want my uterus? "I guess because it's a part of me."

Dr. Jones smiled. "Did you object to having your tonsils removed?"

"That was different. I didn't have much to say about that. I was only six years old."

He was drying his hands now, meticulously. His sunburn gleamed in the early February grayness of a rainy Pacific Northwest afternoon. He threw a sheet over my legs, pulled up a chair, and sat beside me.

"You need a hysterectomy, Naomi. All this heavy bleeding is ridiculous. You shouldn't wait."

I struggled to sit up, was unsuccessful, and sank back down again.

"I don't want surgery," I said firmly. "I've already had five operations on my back. I'm not going through it again."

He lit a cigarette with a gold lighter, leaned back, and took a steadying inhalation of smoke. Exhaling, he said, "I don't know what's wrong with you women. You get so attached to your organs. If I were a woman, I'd not only welcome a hysterectomy, I'd damned well *demand* it after my family had arrived. Who needs all that messy blood every month?"

I finally wrenched myself into a sitting position on the edge of the table with the sheet wrapped firmly around my thighs.

"Yes," he repeated firmly, "after a certain age I'd insist upon a hysterectomy."

"What's a certain age, doctor? I'm not even forty yet. You said yourself I haven't started menopause."

He inhaled again. "Some women start the change of life in their early or mid-thirties. Others not until their late forties or early fifties. Every woman is different. In your case there's no indication that you've started it yet. But that's not the point. You're not planning on having any more children, are you?"

"No, I have my family."

"Then examine the situation realistically. You have your family. You're a very busy woman with a business here in the city to run. Also, I understand that you commute some three hundred miles north to handle the office work for your husband's logging business. In addition to that, you run homes at either end. Can you afford to be knocked out by these bloody messes every three weeks? You tell me you feel exhausted all the time. Can you afford to lose the energy?"

"I'm not arguing with you, doctor. I'm just hoping to find some other answer. Can't you treat me in a way other than surgery?"

I glanced down and gently ran my thumb over the wedding ring my husband had designed for me, with its nineteen diamonds in an unusual pattern. It had always been difficult for me to discuss anything of a sexual nature with anyone, even a doctor. I had always considered sex a highly intimate experience between myself and my lover, to be talked about with absolutely no one. Now, desperation drove me to voice my real fear. I cleared my throat.

"I'm afraid that an operation will affect my sex life."

"Oh, *that's* it!" He laughed richly. "My dear girl, I see that even *you* are a victim of the old wives' tales! Ruin your sex life? No, no, a thousand times no! An operation won't spoil that. It usually makes things better. You can't imagine the number of women who come back after it's all over and tell me, 'Dr. Jones, I had *no idea* sex could be so great!' "

Unable to tune in to his wave of euphoria, I asked how that could be.

"Look, Naomi, I won't be taking out your *sex* organs. I'll be removing your *reproductive* organs. One doesn't have anything to do with the other. You can still taste and enjoy your food, can't you? Having your tonsils out didn't affect *that*. It's the same idea. Your uterus and ovaries have nothing to do with your enjoyment of sex. They're only parts of a baby machine and when you're through making babies they might as well come out. In fact, they *should* come out.

"Now, as far as treating your condition, I could give you a D and C, but that would only be a temporary measure." His silver-framed glasses gleamed in my direction. "You *need* this surgery. You must have this surgery."

He paused as if to allow the thought of what *could* happen to me to sink in. But I'm the sort of person who needs things spelled out. I stared at him, but no further information was forthcoming.

"So what could happen if I just ignore it?" I finally asked.

He leaned forward, tapping my knee with his gold pen. "Do you realize how easy it is for this to become cancerous?"

"Cancer!" I whispered. "You didn't say the tests showed any cancer cells!"

He patted my hand. "They don't—yet. But we doctors see so much of this sort of thing that we can't allow our patients to take chances with their lives. You still have a family to raise and I know your husband wants you around for a good long time. Is a little fear about the quality of your sex life which, I hasten to add, is *entirely* unfounded, worth taking a chance with your whole life?"

"No," I admitted. "No, it isn't."

Then I tried to explain to him how I felt about my uterus. I mean other than its being a part of me. It was where I first nurtured my children, and I also felt that it played an important role in my love life with my husband.

"What's there when you take it away?" I asked.

"You girls and your uteruses." He patted my shoulder jovially. "If you knew more about anatomy you'd realize that the uterus is there for one reason and one reason only, and that's to support and nourish your unborn children. When a woman doesn't want any more children, she has no earthly need for her uterus. Think of it as the nest. The fledglings have flown. *You don't need it anymore.* Every part of your life will be better without it. You'll feel better, you'll be better for your husband and your children. Get rid of it once and for all. Welcome a new and healthy life."

"Maybe I should get another opinion," I ventured.

He removed his glasses and twirled them by the earpiece. "You're certainly welcome to consult whomever you please. All I would ask is that you not wait too long. One of my patients fooled around for six months going from doctor to doctor. Now it's too late. She has inoperable cancer."

I thought for a few minutes. "All right, doctor, you have me convinced. But I want you to leave my cervix and ovaries."

"No way." He rose to his feet. "We'd just be asking for future trouble. When you leave parts of things in it's too easy for them to become cancerous. Trouble with the ovaries is that you can have deeply advanced cancer and not even know it until it's too late. Sorry, I don't work that way. If you want bits and pieces left in, you're perfectly free to go to another gynecologist. After I operate, you won't have to come back for more surgeries. You'll be all through."

How right he was! Eventually, I was all through. But with what, I had yet to learn.

I thought of this man's credentials from local hospitals, from his peers, from the American Medical Association. I had checked up on him. I knew he was considered to be among the best in his field. He had an enormous practice. Who was I to question a professional of such distinction?

"Okay, doctor." I slid off the table ungracefully. "Set it up. I came to you because you're the expert. Advertising is my field. Women's insides is yours."

"Now you're talking." He briskly consulted a file. "Let me see, you just finished a period. Good. Wednesday is my surgery day. Can you be ready next Wednesday, February fourteenth?"

"On Valentine's Day?" Some hearts and flowers for me.

He looked at me blankly. "What difference does it make? You'll be a whole new woman. Your husband will love me when I get your pelvic housecleaning done."

I thought of all the ads I had to create before I could be away for three or four weeks or more. No matter—I would be ready. The specter of cancer had reared its nasty head and I was afraid. I nodded assent.

"I'll want to talk with your husband before surgery." Dr. Jones was already buzzing for his nurse. "Find out when he can come in, then call my west-side office tomorrow morning and arrange it with the receptionist there. She'll pass the word along. Depending on what day your husband can get here, I'll see him either in this office, my Tualatin office, or my downtown office."

I hadn't realized he was running a factory.

I said goodbye, then dashed across Portland to my office to set the crew in motion for twelve full-page color ads for the one client on our list who demanded my personal services. Then I telephoned the client himself, owner of the largest furniture store in the Pacific Northwest and famous all over the country for his aggressive advertising. I told him I would be gone for a month or six weeks because of surgery that could not be delayed. He came right over to the agency.

"Don't worry, I'll have the mechanicals for your ads finished before I leave," I assured him.

11

"In a week? If you can do them that fast I must be paying you too much." He chuckled, then turned serious. "Have you got a good doctor?"

"He's considered one of the five top gynecologists on the west coast."

"Fine. Two things you don't cut costs on are lawyers and doctors," my client advised. "Economize everywhere else, but not there." He rose to leave. "We don't have much time. When do we get together? Tomorrow at eleven in the store?"

"Tomorrow at eleven," I agreed.

That night I worked late. I wouldn't be able to reach my husband in Moclips (on the Olympic Peninsula) until long after dark, when he had come in out of the woods. Then his phone would be ringing off the hook. Loggers confine their business to the nighttime hours when they can't work outside.

I left the agency about nine, stopped for a quick meal at a restaurant, then went home, took a hot shower, picked up a book, and collapsed into bed. Around eleven I got through to Joe.

"Hi, honey, it's me. What's going on up there in the forest primeval?"

"Had a hell of a storm blow up." Joe's voice rumbled four hundred miles down the line. "If this wind doesn't let up, the crews won't be able to work tomorrow. Too dangerous." There was a pause, then his voice came back on the line. "Good God, the spray from the waves is drenching the front windows. The ocean must be ten feet deep at our retaining wall."

"Go up to the hotel on the cliff," I urged. "A heavy storm could sweep the house right off that bank. Take Matt and Meg and go. I don't want to worry about you, too."

"If it gets much worse, we will. The kids are sound asleep. I hate to disturb them." There was silence for a moment. "What do you mean, worry about us, *too?* What else are you worrying about down there? Honey? Did you go to the doctor today?"

"Yes," I sighed.

"Well? What did he say?"

"He said I've got to have a hysterectomy!" I burst out. "I

don't want to but he says I can't put it off. He wants to talk to you as soon as you can get down here. He's going to operate next Wednesday!" I wailed.

"Take it easy, honey." Joe's voice was calm. "We'll take off first thing in the morning. It won't hurt the kids to miss a day or so at school. Now go to sleep and get some rest. I love you, honey. You're going to be all right. Remember that."

How I wanted my husband that night. I longed to snuggle in his arms and go to sleep, although snuggling meant *not* going to sleep right away.

I had been married before. I had always found the sexual experience rewarding but never, in the wildest flights of my imagination, did I ever think it could be the superb physical pleasure I had found in this marriage. Even a glance across the room would set us wanting each other. After four years of marriage, our happiness in each other had in no way dimmed.

When Joe and I had married, I had recently concluded a hopeless marriage and he had been single for thirteen years. He adopted my four children. We were indeed a family. I thought of the two younger children coming home from school not long before and telling me how sorry they felt for their friends because in the entire room they were the only ones with their *real* Mom and Dad. Our love was so strong that Matt and Meg had actually forgotten that Joe was not their real father. What we had all found in each other we didn't think existed outside of books.

And what Joe and I had found in our lovemaking was almost beyond understanding. *Please God,* I prayed, *don't let it be spoiled.*

When Joe and I came out of Dr. Jones's office the next day, my husband's normally ruddy outdoor complexion was pale. We got into the car without saying anything. Before he started the engine, I asked, "Should I put it off?"

"God, no! We can't waste a day. I tried to talk the Doc into doing it sooner. But next Wednesday it is."

"It isn't any worse than I think, is it?" I asked slowly. "You'd tell me the truth, wouldn't you? I don't care what it is, it's always easier to deal with the truth."

He slammed the gearshift into park, then turned and grabbed me in his arms. "Honey, you know the whole story. Doc Jones didn't hold anything back. But, my God, you're on the verge of something that could be disastrous. You can't play around with this thing. You've got to go through with it. I couldn't live if anything happened to you."

"But how can I be on the verge of cancer? I thought one either had cancer or didn't have it. I don't understand this at all . . ."

"We're not taking any chances with your life. Let's go home and be by ourselves. Mindy's going to keep Matt and Meg on the campus with her this evening. I've got to be back up on the peninsula in the morning. Got some timber buyers coming. Can't you get someone else to do those ads? Come back up north with me until you have to go into the hospital?"

"I can't. My touch is what this client is paying for. I'll have to work straight through the weekend. But that's good. It'll keep my mind off what's coming next week."

"I'll be back the day before you go in. Sooner, if possible." Joe reached over and took my hand. "You've got to be checked into Good Sam by three. If I know you, you'll work right up until two thirty. I'll be here to see that you get there on time, if nothing else." He gave me his big white-toothed grin that I loved.

"Won't you be here the night before? I was hoping we'd spend that last night together."

"You know I will, sweetheart."

We looked at each other for a long time. Then he said softly, "Let's go home."

Neither of us slept much that night. It was as if we didn't want to waste a moment in the unconsciousness of sleep.

As I went about my work at the advertising agency, my mind was full of the coming surgery. Something deep inside whispered: *Don't have that operation. Refuse. You don't need it.*

14

I reached for the phone to call Dr. Jones. In business I invariably made mistakes when I didn't follow my instincts. But this wasn't business. This could be my *life*. How could I, who knew nothing about my body, dispute a prominent physician whose lifework was treating women?

Still the inner voice persisted: *You don't need the operation. So you bleed a little heavily. That won't kill you.*

But it might, I thought. It just might. Dr. Jones had intimated to me, and had told Joe more directly, that what I had could quickly turn into cancer.

Maybe I already had cancer. Maybe Dr. Jones and my husband were protecting me from devastating knowledge.

I had been brought up to revere the medical profession. In the church I belonged to as a child, parents hoped that their sons and daughters would become doctors and nurses and medical missionaries. Doctors were good. In fact, I remembered one pastor saying that doctors were God's hands on earth.

You don't need that operation. . . . But the inner voice was fainter now, as if it were going away.

Dr. Jones was a fine doctor. His wall was covered with diplomas and awards. I would do the right thing. I would have the surgery.

On the morning of Valentine's Day, February 14, I lay on my hospital bed listening to a savage Pacific storm beat against the windows of my room.

For that first night and the first day after surgery, I would have to share a room with two other women; the private room I had requested wouldn't be available for a couple of days. The occupant of the bed next to mine had been given her pre-op shots about six in the morning. She seemed nearly comatose. The lady across the room had undergone surgery the day before and was still out of it. Essentially I was alone in the early morning dimness.

Joe had come down from the Olympic Peninsula the day before yesterday, but he had contracted such a severe case of flu that he wanted to stay as far away from me as possible.

"It isn't going to help you if you get the flu just before the operation," he said as he headed down the hall toward one of the guest rooms in our Portland home. "I'm sorry, honey, this isn't the way I'd planned on spending this night."

The day before I had worked until 2:45 in the afternoon. I wanted to take a cab to the hospital since Joe was in such bad shape. But he insisted on taking me there himself. He was carrying a small overnight case and three shopping bags full of books I intended to read during my stay.

During the early evening my daughter Mindy arrived from her classes at Lewis & Clark College. A couple of friends dropped by, too.

Everyone, including the nurses, thought it was hilarious that I had brought so many books. "Mom's a reader," Mindy explained. "She can't do without her books."

Soon they all prepared to go. Joe blew me a kiss and assured me he'd be back in the morning. I knew if he hadn't been feeling so rotten he would have stayed with me until lights out.

I stretched out on the bed and read. My reading was interrupted periodically by nurses taking blood, the staff intern getting information for the hospital records, and the anesthesiologist coming in for a chat. Dr. Jones popped in briefly and stood by my bed.

"All set?" he asked, eyes twinkling behind polished lenses.

"I guess so. I just didn't want to have a hysterectomy this young."

He leaned down to whisper. "Young? That gal next to you is only twenty-four. She can't wait to get rid of the stuff. After tomorrow she won't have to worry about getting pregnant anymore."

He straightened, waved, and called out that he'd see me in the morning around ten, in surgery. Then he was gone, leaving an after-image of expensive cologne, gleaming teeth and shiny glasses.

It was all very cheery and comforting. I felt as if I were joining a select group. Most important of all, I felt surrounded by caring experts who were holding the outside world at bay.

Around ten o'clock I was led down the hall for a shower, and at about ten-thirty the "prepper" arrived with razor, lather, and bowl. A few minutes after eleven the medicine nurse on the new shift came around with a shot to put me to sleep.

As I drifted off, I began to think Dr. Jones was right. After tomorrow, no more messy menstruation. Soon I would be free of all that.

And now the morning was here. Valentine's Day. Someone had brought in a big box of candy. There was a muted bustle in the hall as the lucky ones were served breakfast trays. I would have given my right arm for a cup of hot black coffee.

Joe arrived looking sick. Mindy bustled in, telling me she had cut all her classes this day so she could be with me. I told her she wouldn't see much of me and what she saw wouldn't be conversational.

"That's okay, Mom." She kissed me. "I'm going to be here. I don't care how long it takes."

Around nine, a nurse brought in the first shot, which left me relaxed, and about half an hour later she came back in with the second shot. In a few minutes my mouth was so dry it was difficult to talk. No water was allowed. Joe held one hand, Mindy the other. I felt like I'd like to stay that way forever.

"Mrs. Stokes?" The questioning voice was male. I opened my eyes and saw a blur of green in the doorway. It seemed that a couple of young men had arrived to take me somewhere, I wasn't sure where. One was slender, short, and dark. The other was plump and massive. They rolled a gurney to the side of my bed, threw my covers back, smoothed my hospital gown and slid me expertly onto the rolling table. Joe cupped my face with his hands, Mindy gave me another soft kiss, and I was off.

We traveled to the elevator, descended somewhere into the bowels of the earth, traversed an underground passageway, then rolled into another elevator. Then there was a hallway from which a series of brightly lighted rooms branched off. Somewhere I could hear a radio playing softly. A couple of people came by to verify that I was indeed Naomi Stokes. A nurse bent over me.

"Your operating room will be ready in a few minutes, Mrs. Stokes. They're just finishing up a lady in there now."

Finishing up a lady? My thoughts were wild and confused. Poor lady, does she know she's being finished up? *Stop it! You've got to stay awake long enough to talk to the anesthesiologist.* I dozed for a while and then came to again as I felt the gurney rolling.

"Can you slide over on the table, Mrs. Stokes?"

"Sure," I mumbled. "I can do anything. All you have to do is ask."

Then I was on the operating table, trying to clear my eyes enough to take in my surroundings. It's difficult to see or make sense of what you're seeing after prep-op shots. I felt myself being strapped down and sensed activity at my head, beyond my sight.

"Is that the anesthesiologist?" I forced my voice out.

"It's me, Mrs. Stokes," came a cheerful voice. A green-shrouded figure appeared on my right. "I'm going to put this needle in your vein and when we're ready for the anesthetic you won't even know it."

I licked my dry lips with a flannel tongue. "Please tell me when. Please don't knock me out until you tell me when you're going to. Please."

He patted my hand. "Sure enough. I'll tell you first and then I'll have you start counting backward from one hundred."

I could hear the clatter of pans and the soft squeaky-swish of the nurses' shoes. I felt I was sinking, sinking . . . I pulled myself awake abruptly.

"Is the doctor here yet?"

"Not yet," one of the nurses replied. "Should be any minute now."

There was a bustle, then Dr. Jones's voice called out, "Hi, gang. All set?" I sensed that he was joking with the nurses but I couldn't quite make out what he was saying.

Suddenly he loomed over me, a massive greenness broken

only by a suntanned piece of face and those perpetually gleaming glasses. "Ah, there you are, Naomi. How are you feeling?"

"Scared." The word whispered out over cracked lips. Tears blurred my eyes. "I'm scared. Let me hold your hand."

"I'm sorry, dear, but I'm sterile." He held up his gloved hands.

I will be soon, too. Then the thought whisked itself away.

Don't let them do it, the inner voice whispered.

The glasses glistened in my direction again. "What?" He bent over me. Then he raised up and I heard him say, "Go."

The anesthesiologist's voice came clear and masculine and soft. "We're ready now, Mrs. Stokes. I'm going to start the anesthesia. Just start counting backward from one hundred please . . ."

"No. No, wait! I'm not ready!" I thought I screamed it out. They told me later that I had said nothing.

". . . now, Mrs. Stokes, one hundred . . . ninety-nine . . . ninety-eight . . ."

I was deep within myself, perhaps five hundred miles down at least.

I felt attached to something, a body, perhaps, but it didn't feel like mine. There was the beginning of nausea, but it was someone else's nausea and I couldn't figure out how *I* was feeling it. Me, the real me, sank even deeper into a depthless pool. I could just barely hear a woman's voice. It seemed that she was calling from a long way off.

"Mrs. Stokes!" the voice cried. "Mrs. Stokes, wake up, Mrs. Stokes!"

Stop that yelling, I thought. I tried to let her know I was all right so she wouldn't worry but I couldn't make anything work in this strange body. I tried to open its eyes and its mouth to whisper that I was okay, but the body wasn't obeying.

I sank deeper, further away. The nurse was doing something to the body's arm, but I didn't care. I wanted to be left alone. Then I heard her voice again, shouting down a tunnel this time.

19

"Better call the doctor. She doesn't have any pressure. I can't get any pressure at all."

Another woman's voice joined hers and I heard the bark of authority. "Mrs. Stokes!" it commanded. "Mrs. Stokes! You've got to wake up. Now, Mrs. Stokes. Wake up!"

By then I had figured out the body wasn't responding because it wasn't mine. I couldn't understand why these women were so stupid they were calling a strange body by my name and expecting it to obey.

"Mrs. Stokes!" I heard slapping sounds and felt jars and thuds as if the body were being vigorously slapped.

Where are you, my children? I thought, then sank deeper yet. And kept on sinking until I sank right down to my small girlhood. *Mother! Daddy! Where are you?* And then I sank into darkness so deep there was nothing there, not even the past.

My next awareness was ghastly tearing pain in my abdomen as I heaved painfully. I felt cold metal against my cheek.

"God," I groaned. "Help me. I'm coming apart."

"Try not to vomit, Mrs. Stokes," came a female voice. "We're giving you a shot to stop that nausea."

Another horrible retch overcame me. The result of gigantic stomach heaves was an unrewarding dribble in the emesis basin. I could feel my eyelids opening but I couldn't see anything.

"Where am I?" I whispered.

"In the recovery room," came a brisk voice. "Just cooperate with us now and we'll have you back in your room in no time."

What am I supposed to do? I wondered. *I'm not even sure who I am.*

"Keep awake, Mrs. Stokes, keep awake. That will help your blood pressure come back up."

I heard the slapping sounds again. "Come on now, don't go back to sleep."

I started to sink again. Then, suddenly, I soared out of the depths. I couldn't see, but I knew I was in the recovery room.

I heard the rustle of bedclothes being pulled back, then a different voice telling me it was giving me a shot.

"You'll feel something cold, Mrs. Stokes, then just a pinprick."

I lost consciousness again, but didn't sink into that terrifying blackness. Sometime later I awoke, and opened my eyes to a dazzling white room. Instantly I heard the squish of a nurse's shoes and there was a white presence beside me.

"Welcome back, Mrs. Stokes," a pleasant voice said. "You had us a little worried there for awhile." She vanished.

Then, after another long period of blankness, a sharp voice said, "Cough, Mrs. Stokes, cough! You've got to cough!"

I lay there like a log. Cough? She must be mad! I couldn't cough. I'd tear out my stitches. Didn't she know I'd just had surgery?

"Mrs. Stokes." This time the voice brooked no disobedience. I felt hands on my chest. "Cough! Cough! Now! That's it. Now keep at it until you get some fluid up." I tried valiantly. "Fine, that's fine. Here, spit it out."

I lay back exhausted. I heard the nurse say, "We've got to do that every twenty minutes right through the night."

My right hand was being squeezed and massaged and then held almost with desperation. Then Mindy's voice came, sounding like it had when she was a little girl.

"Mom, are you all right?"

"Fine, honey. Don't worry."

Will she ever know how much I love her, I wondered. I just want her to be happy. I drifted off.

The night was a delirium of nausea, extreme pain, and demands that I cough.

The next day, I was moved into my private room. Around eleven in the morning, as I lay there staring down at my body stretched long and straight under the covers, my furniture store client arrived.

"What have they done to you?" he asked, walking around the bed.

"They've turned me into a boy," I replied.

Then I was asleep again. Later in the day a woman friend came with gifts. "You'll be just fine," she said. "I know. I went through this ten years ago. The best part is that things won't bother you as much as they did before. Hysterectomy has a very calming effect."

"That's exactly the effect it had on my beagle," I murmured. "She changed from a high-spirited pup into a stuffy matron, all with a few strokes of the scalpel."

I thought I was kidding.

For the next few days convalescence progressed unremarkably. On the fourth day, I got out of bed to go to the bathroom. A bright red flood gushed down my legs. The young nurse who was helping me froze. I shook her off and got to the toilet where I sat down, pulled my gown up and saw immediately that the blood was coming from the external incision rather than from an internal hemorrhage.

"It's all right," I called to her. "The incision just opened up. Get somebody."

She was gone in a blur, but returned almost immediately with the head nurse. They helped me back to bed, examined the opening wound, left to call the doctor, returned with the "medicine girl" who rebandaged me tightly. Then they gave me a shot to calm me, although I was the calmest in the group.

The days passed. I read. Company came. Television was boring. Flowers arrived. The telephone rang. I was healing.

During one of Dr. Jones's visits I asked what happened to the space that was left after the organs came out.

He laughed. "Everybody wonders about that. The other stuff in there just sort of moves around and fills it up. There's a lot of empty space inside a human body. Our various organs aren't packed in that tightly. If they were, it would be disastrous when we fill up with gas."

Grinning, he left. For the past few days I'd had the feeling that I was history to Dr. Jones. He had taken his pound of flesh. I was recuperating. Of what further interest could I be to him? My thoughts turned vigorously to getting out of there.

When the time came, I was more than ready to go. I had stayed two weeks because there was no one to take care of me in our Portland home. Also, the home was built on a series of levels which would be difficult for me to negotiate.

I wanted to spend my recovery with my husband up in the logging country. Dr. Jones said there was no way he would let me make a five-hour trip unless it was by ambulance. When Joe explained that the thick foam seats in his car reclined fully, that in effect I'd be lying down, Dr. Jones gave his permission.

The day of departure was clear and bright. I dressed in a tailored suit and was ceremoniously wheeled to the waiting car. I had a full supply of Percodan for pain, hydrogen peroxide to keep the surgical wound clean, and various bandages.

It felt so good to be out in the air, I wanted to run around the block. That lasted for two seconds. By the time I stood up from the wheelchair I was ready to stretch out in the comfortable car bed.

At the halfway point to Moclips, we stopped at an excellent restaurant. What a relief from the hospital offerings! Then I stretched out in the Citroen again and when I awoke, we were turning into our driveway at the beach. Joe helped me out and I stood propped up by the car for long minutes just breathing that wonderful fragrance of salt spray, wood smoke, wind gusting in from the Pacific Ocean, and fir and cedar incense from the great timber stands. What a place to get well!

Matt and Meg came tearing out of the house, all loving concern and wet kisses. I must hurry in to eat the special chocolate pudding they'd made for me. And then there was David, my firstborn, with the smile that remained from boyhood, the smile that said, "Mom, you're special to me."

He enfolded me in his arms. "Hi, Mom. I've been worried about you. But with Dad gone I couldn't leave the woods. Are you okay now?"

With David the message is always in the eyes. I looked deep into his sparkling blue ones and knew I was all right, I was fine, now that I was with most of my family. (Mindy had remained at college in Portland.)

So, home to the woods, with the surf crashing and the sea gulls crying and most of my loves about me. I needed to get right into bed, which I did. Then I ate my pudding, held all their hands, and fell asleep thinking, *Was ever a woman so blessed?*

Each day I did a little more. I would rise to prepare a meal, watch the ocean, walk a bit, then lie down for several hours. I read incessantly and at night I slept in Joe's arms.

I longed to walk on the beach in the spring storms but I wasn't yet up to climbing up and down the bank. Joe promised that after we got back from Portland for my month's checkup he'd lift me up and down and walk with me.

I noticed that after I was on my feet for ten or fifteen minutes I experienced lightning-like flashes of "bright pain" running diagonally deep down in my abdomen. It caused me some alarm, even though I associated the pain with the final healing of severed parts. The rusty vaginal discharge was nearly gone.

Other than that, the most I felt was a certain "emptiness" in the abdominal area, not like a great empty space, but a space empty of feeling. I had always been able to feel my uterus.

A heavy March storm was blowing up the morning we left Moclips for the journey to Portland. I sat up all the way with three or four breaks to stretch my legs and have coffee.

When we arrived in Dr. Jones's office, his waiting room was crowded as usual. Because of the distance we had traveled, Dr. Jones had instructed the receptionist to work me in between other patients as soon as I arrived. I appreciated his consideration. I had been sitting in the car for nearly five hours.

Dr. Jones ushered me into an examining room, left momentarily while I took off my clothes and put on the paper gown. When he returned, he conducted the examination. His fingers were gentle but his speculum was cold.

"Healing beautifully," he pronounced.

I told him about the flashes of "bright pain."

"What's bright pain?"

"It's like a lightning flash, only instead of light, it's pain."

"Are you sure you're not a poet?" He favored me with his

widest smile. "Don't worry about it. Now I've got great news for you."

This time he helped me into a sitting position on the end of the examining table. "Remember your worries about sex after the operation?" I was nearly blinded by the combined sparkle from his glasses and his teeth. "Well, tonight's the night. I want you to have sex with your husband."

I was stunned. Sex on command? Women are usually advised to abstain from sex for six weeks after childbirth. This was only one month after surgery.

"Suppose something breaks?" I asked.

"For heaven's sake, do you think I'd recommend it if I thought it would be harmful in any way? Don't be silly."

By the time I got out of the doctor's office, I was extremely nauseated and felt like I was going to faint. I also felt a discharge although that was probably caused by the examination.

Joe and I stopped at a restaurant for an early dinner. The food made me feel somewhat better, but I still needed to get to our Portland home and lie down.

"Dr. Jones said we should make love tonight," I announced.

Joe looked at me in disbelief. "Do you feel like it? You know I'd never touch you unless you wanted it as much as I did."

I toyed with my coffee cup. "He didn't actually say we should make love. He prescribed sex like a medication. No, I don't feel like it yet but he said it's important that we don't wait."

"We'll just forget it until you're ready." Joe lit his pipe.

I'd had visions of going to a movie or doing something in the city but we were both exhausted. We went home (which seemed dreary and impersonal with all the family gone), showered, and fell into bed.

As we lay in each other's arms, I whispered, "I think we should try. He said it was important to my recovery."

I could feel Joe smiling in the darkness. "I don't need a second invitation."

But it was too painful.

"I'm sorry, honey," I murmured. "Maybe there's something wrong with me."

Looking back, I realize that was the first time I felt guilty about there "being something wrong with me" since I'd had the surgery. It would not be the last time.

"Call that doctor in the morning and see what he has to say," Joe told me. "We'll stay another day if we have to."

I fell into a troubled sleep. There had been absolutely no stirring of desire when my husband's hands touched me. Of course, I *was* overly tired. And I *was* just one month out of surgery. Things would get better.

In the morning Dr. Jones purred a greeting over the telephone, then paused as I told him about my troubles.

"That's nothing to worry about," he consoled. "I didn't really think things would work right yet but I wanted you to get in there and try. It's like falling off a horse. You've got to get right back on."

Falling off a horse?

"Just think of all the fun you'll have trying," he went on.

Fun?

"But I didn't feel anything except pain," I protested.

"That's all right." He chuckled. "Maybe your husband's a little more of a man than others. Tell him to take it easy, and hang in there."

The line went dead. I was beginning to actively dislike Dr. Jones.

We returned to our home by the sea. Joe was in the woods from before daybreak until long after dark. One night I woke up crying.

"What is it, honey?" Joe cuddled me in his arms.

"Make love to me," I sobbed.

"Are you sure? I've had the feeling lately that you'd rather just be left alone." He was silent for a time. "Do I turn you off?"

I put my hand on him gently. "It isn't you, Joe, it's me. I don't know what's wrong."

"I thought you'd gotten tired of me. People sometimes do, you know. Get tired of each other. But I can't complain. It was wonderful while it lasted."

"Oh, Joe, I'm not tired of you. Never tired of you. I can't explain how I feel. Or don't feel."

"It isn't any good if we force it, honey."

I could feel anger growing. He was the nearest target. "Don't you understand?" I shouted. "I *have* to force it. That's the only way I can do anything. And then it isn't any good for me."

How can he be so stupid, I thought. If he really loved me, he'd know how I feel. I had yet to learn how much damage that attitude can do to a relationship. A man's love is not a guarantee that he's a mind reader, that he automatically knows your innermost feelings.

But I didn't know that then. I also didn't know that the medical experts were wrong, those experts who were telling women that there is nothing about a hysterectomy that can cause crippling sexual difficulties.

"Just forget it," I muttered. "It's a sorry day when I have to ask a man to make love to me."

Time went by. I visited Dr. Jones several times, talking to him about my problem. He seemed as puzzled as I although it was apparent he didn't take my complaint seriously. He gave me the name of a clinical psychologist with whom I made an appointment. I went to him for five sessions. None of what he said made sense in my situation.

I went to the Multnomah County Public Library, considered one of the finest libraries in the country, and read everything I could lay my hands on about hysterectomy and its possible effect on sexuality. Nothing. Oh, the subject was mentioned but only in regard to a few odd women whose complaints were "definitely psychological in origin."

I went back to see Dr. Jones. "Could I talk with some of your patients who've told you how much better sex is after hysterectomy?" I asked.

He pondered my question gravely. "There's really no way I could intrude on their privacy."

He must have sensed my determination because he quickly added, "Of course, I could give a couple of them your name and number and suggest they call you."

Weeks passed. I did not hear from any of Dr. Jones's happy patients. Perhaps they were all too busy in bed.

One night Joe came home late from a meeting in the bar at the hotel on the cliff. "I've heard everything now," he laughed. "You know Sam Jackson, the judge on the Quinault Indian reservation?"

I nodded.

"He was telling me tonight that he's hearing a case for divorce tomorrow. Old Man Miller's wife had a hysterectomy and his charge against her is that she can't have any more kids."

"Any *more?* He's got eighteen."

"Yeah. But he says his daddy had twenty and it's always been his ambition to have twenty kids, too, just like his pa. He's already got one of the young Indian gals picked out to replace Ida."

"Will Sam give him a divorce?" I knew the Indians had their own laws on the reservation and the white man couldn't intrude. "And what about the Indian girl? What young girl would want to marry an old man like that?"

"Old? He's only fifty." Was Joe's voice a little defensive? *He* was only fifty. "Sam's going to give him the divorce. He says Miller's entitled to as many kids as he wants. The young gal is rarin' to go. Miller's got a lot of timber holdings. I'm sure she's looking at the money." Joe pulled off his boots. "The judge says after an operation like that a woman's never what she used to be. But he'll see that Miller leaves the first wife well fixed."

Joe didn't realize what he'd said. I walked over to poke the fire and hide my tears. Maybe the Indians knew more than the doctors.

I began to wonder about myself. Perhaps I was getting tired of my husband. Maybe I didn't want to admit it but my body was admitting it for me. Or, maybe I was getting old. Old? At forty? Maybe I should take a lover. That should prove once and for all whether I still had the old sparkle. I knew a lot of men, but none of them looked as good to me as my own husband.

Then another thought surfaced, and I began to doubt my own sexuality, to question my interest in men. Had I, in the course of an hour's surgery, become asexual? What was happening to me?

My body remained quiet. I began to look at my husband with a critical eye. Maybe it was his fault. Maybe I was tired of his exuberance. Ah, but I adored his exuberance! It was the second main reason I had married him. He was so *alive.*

Maybe he was too sharp with the kids now and then. But the two youngest were approaching their teen years and needed a firm hand. Besides, he loved them. He had always thanked me for bringing four such wonderful children to our marriage.

Maybe he didn't give me enough tenderness. But since the operation I had turned him away consistently. He was not the sort of man who used a woman as a convenience.

Maybe he had a lover. But when? We were almost always together. But were we? What about all those weeks when I was in Portland and he was up in the woods? Absolutely ridiculous, I thought. He's not a cheat. But didn't he always say that good sex was 98 percent of a good marriage? How long had it been since I'd heard him say *that?*

I would have given almost anything to recover the priceless old spontaneity of days gone by.

A year passed. Then another. Still I had no sexual desire. I had used up all the excuses, gone from doctor to doctor, consulted several psychologists and a psychiatrist. Nothing. My body was a barren field, bereft of the joy of anticipation. I could remember the passion but I could no longer summon it.

A distance had formed between my husband and myself, manifesting itself in a certain coolness in greeting, certain long silences when we were together. We no longer touched. When we went to bed at night, we turned to our books instead of to each other. Sadly I remembered the days when dinner had to wait, when it was torture to be apart for one night. Now it didn't matter. The bedroom door that used to be locked a lot now stood ajar.

Dr. Jones had a long talk with Joe in private. Later I heard about their conversation. The doctor told Joe that whatever was wrong with me had absolutely nothing to do with the hysterectomy.

"The problem is within your marriage," he said. "I've run into this before. Women whose marriages are in trouble like to blame their operations."

"But there was no trouble before the operation," Joe said.

"There had to be. Trouble that you didn't know about."

"What kind of trouble?"

"Who knows?" The doctor had shaken his head. "Hysterectomy is the most maligned operation I know of."

"You mean other women have complained? My wife's been reading whatever she can find and everything says sex is better afterward."

Dr. Jones nodded. "That's the way it should be. But women are always complaining. For one thing, when women have this kind of surgery they're usually not in the first flush of youth. And, my God, as soon as they have a hysterectomy they start having problems in bed. It's ridiculous. All I can say is there's a certain 'lunatic fringe,' if you'll pardon the expression, that makes this kind of complaint."

Joe told me he had to restrain himself from hitting Dr. Jones.

Our lives went on but the zest was gone. I told Joe I wanted a divorce. I didn't want to live with him anymore. Privately I saw him as a constant reminder of my sexual loss. He suggested waiting before a final decision was reached. I perceived him as my enemy instead of as my lover and my friend. A great depression fell over me. I thought of suicide.

During the years I had run the advertising agency I had

periodically written and published articles on various subjects. My dream was to eventually write full time and, in anticipation of this, I began attending authors' seminars. During one such function I met a marriage counselor and sex therapist who told me that 98 percent of her patients were women with extreme sexual difficulties following hysterectomy.

For the first time in four years I brightened. Perhaps I wasn't the freak I thought myself to be. I went to a different gynecologist, Dr. George Hara, who had delivered my two youngest children. Due to conflicting time schedules, I had not consulted him for the surgery I had undergone. Now I invoked the bond of old friendship.

"Please get my records from Dr. Jones," I asked him. "And please look them over."

One week later I was back in Dr. Hara's office.

"We can't reverse anything, Naomi," he said slowly.

"I know that. I also know it would be easier for both of us for you to tell me that I absolutely had to have that hysterectomy. But I beg you to tell me the truth, whatever the truth is. What would you have done given the condition my medical records show?"

For a few moments there was silence as he studied the folder containing my medical records. All around his office walls were photographic studies, evidence of his favorite hobby. I remembered that when my youngest child was born, Dr. Hara told me he had taken up obstetrics because it was such a happy practice. Most of the children he delivered were eagerly awaited by loving parents.

Now he looked at me carefully before replying. "Okay, Naomi, here it is." He glanced again at the open folder. "First of all, your condition as shown here should have been thoroughly discussed with you. I believe it could have been successfully treated with hormone therapy. Personally, I don't think you should have had the surgery."

Hearing this, I felt unnaturally composed, beyond anger, as if it were all merely a dream.

He bent again to the records. " 'Pelvic housecleaning,' " he murmured. "What a terrible phrase. Makes it sound like a woman's insides are garbage."

"Are you aware that Dr. Jones did my surgery on Valentine's Day?"

Again, Dr. Hara shook his head. "Maybe he doesn't believe in hearts and flowers." He looked at me doubtfully. "I'm truly sorry, Naomi. But you asked me to tell you the truth."

"Yes," I said calmly. "I needed to know. Now I realize what I have to do."

"And what is that?"

"I'm going to interview as many women as I can find who have had hysterectomies and discover for myself if what I suspect is really true."

"What do you suspect?"

"That a complete hysterectomy kills sexual desire. If what I find will save just one woman from this experience, the effort will be well worth it."

"That would be fascinating research. Please keep me informed."

"Women are entitled to know the truth," I went on. "My marriage has deteriorated to a couple of strangers living in the same house. How many other women like that are out there? Even if my operation had been necessary for life-saving reasons, I still should have been told the truth about it."

"If you had known it would harm your sexuality you might not have permitted the surgery."

"As it turns out, I seem not to have needed it," I replied. "A woman is entitled to know the possibilities. For women who must have the surgery, maybe there could be some sort of counseling or sex therapy that she and her husband could be made aware of. Anyway," I rose to leave, "whatever the truth is, I'm going to find it."

And so began my search.

Chapter One

HYSTERECTOMY:
THE UNKINDEST
CUT OF ALL

Hysterectomy is the most frequently performed major surgery in the United States.

It has become a growth industry, a very big business, with over $1.7 billion spent each year on the surgical procedure alone. The medical profession assures us that hysterectomy will continue to be an important part of the health care of American women in the years ahead. Which is very bad news, indeed.

The cost to women in terms of physiological and sexual dysfunction is staggering. Tragically, well over 90 percent of these operations are clearly unnecessary. Most of them could have been avoided by the use of alternative therapy. Many are done for downright foolish reasons. Of all the hysterectomies performed each year, about one out of five is for sterilization only, with absolutely no legitimate medical reason.

One of the most stunning aspects of this needless butchery is that the medical profession's marvelous new microsurgery techniques, the development of plastic surgery, ultrasound, and new knowledge about hormones actually make most of these surgeries unnecessary.

How prevalent is this blight? During the nine-year period from 1970 to 1978, approximately 3,536,000 young women between the ages of 14 and 44 had hysterectomies. In 1980, American physicians performed 649,000 reported hysterectomies. In 1981, the figure rose to 673,000 and dropped in 1982 to 650,000. In 1983 it soared to a whopping 672,000. Approximately one-half of all hysterectomies involve removal of the patient's ovaries.

These figures do not include women undergoing hysterectomy in federally operated hospitals, such as Armed Forces and Public Health Service hospitals, nor do they include the number of women who have undergone radical hysterectomy (removal of uterus, cervix, tubes, ovaries, adjacent lymph glands, and part of the vagina) or pelvic exenterations (even more radical removal of the lower bodily cavity such as all of the vagina and part of the bowel). Total number of hysterectomies done each year is conservatively estimated at over one million.

Women usually refer to the operation as being a "complete" hysterectomy, by which they mean the removal of the uterus, tubes, and ovaries. In medical terms, if both the Fallopian tubes and ovaries are removed, the operation is correctly called a total hysterectomy and bilateral (both sides) salpingo-oophorectomy (tubes and ovaries removed). It is a surgery that has been subjected to intense scrutiny in recent years by consumer groups, government agencies, insurance companies, and professional societies. Almost no one has spoken for the women who undergo the operation.

Hysterectomy is one of several surgical procedures which threaten human sexuality. Others are the "ostomies"—colostomy, cystostomy, and ileostomy. Colostomy is the formation of a surgical fistula, or opening, which periodically voids fecal matter from the large intestine into a bag. Cystostomy is a surgical opening from the bladder which voids into a bag. Ileostomy is the formation of a surgical opening from the small intestine which drains continuously into a bag.

These are difficult surgeries. They have a dramatic effect on sexuality for both women and men. But hysterectomy represents a special peril all its own. One does not wear an external bag after the surgery. One need not fear the odor from escaping body fluids. The aftermath of hysterectomy for many women is much worse. They are left with anaphrodisia, or loss of sexual desire and feeling.

The truth is that an appalling subculture of American women suffer in silence from a loss of sexual desire, or libido, as a result of this surgery. Whatever it is called, the result is the same. Women no longer have any desire to have sex with their husbands or lovers. The loss is not limited to heterosexual sex. Lesbian women report the same problem and are given the usual medical double talk and shuffled off for psychoanalysis.

"Don't worry about sex," said one doctor. "Hysterectomy isn't any worse than having your tonsils out."

Hysterectomy is much worse than having one's tonsils out. Research shows it is a surgery that wreaks far-reaching havoc, of which sexual dysfunction may be only one result.

A relatively new finding is that the hormonal changes brought about by hysterectomy frequently result in atherosclerotic heart disease. Four independent investigations have shown a threefold increase in such heart disease following hysterectomy. It is thought that prostacyclin, a potent vasodilator and inhibitor of platelet aggregation produced by the uterus, protects women who still have their uteruses from heart failure.

Another serious side effect is posthysterectomy syndrome, a nicer term for severe suicidal depression. Hysterectomy patients have double the number of postoperative admissions to psychiatric hospitals as do patients who have undergone other kinds of surgery. It is noteworthy that these patients have an important *lack* of prior psychiatric history.

The third side effect is the one talked about the least—the one thought for years to be nothing more than "old wives' tales" or sick fantasies indulged in by half-crazy menopausal women. This side effect has to do with the most intimate part of a woman's life—her sexuality.

Every woman faces the possibility that hysterectomy will be recommended at some time during her life. According to the figures, this will happen during her young womanhood. A detailed analysis performed by the National Center for Health

Statistics (NCHS) reveals that in 1978, for example, 63 percent of the women who underwent this operation were 15 to 44 years old, 31 percent were 45 to 64 years old, and only six percent were 65 or older.

In the United States the majority of hysterectomies are performed upon women during their reproductive years. Perhaps this is why approximately 27 percent of the women in this country of childbearing age can have no children. [This figure does not include women who are infertile.] According to a report from the NCHS, of the 54 million women between the ages of 15 and 44, almost 9.5 million have chosen to be sterilized for reasons of birth control. An additional 4.2 million have been surgically sterilized for other reasons. And 4.4 million are so physically handicapped that conception and successful pregnancy would be either extremely difficult or downright impossible. According to the National Center, sterilization by surgery is the leading method of birth control in the United States. An appalling number of these sterilizations have been accomplished by hysterectomy.

American women know the inside of operating rooms far too well. Of the ten most frequently performed surgical procedures, five are performed solely for women. According to the American College of Surgeons, the list of the ten most frequently performed surgeries (based on 1980 figures) are as follows:

Biopsy (surgical removal of tissue to determine diagnosis)	1,535,000
Dilation and currettage (D and C)	923,000
Excisions of lesions on skin or tissue	715,000
Hysterectomy	649,000
Ligation and division of fallopian tubes	641,000
Cesarean section	619,000
Hernia repair	537,000
Oophorectomy (ovary removal)	483,000
Cataract removal	467,000
Removal of tonsils and adenoids	464,000

Of all the adult women in the country today, 62 percent will have had a hysterectomy (removal of the uterus) and/or oophorectomy (removal of the ovaries) by the time they are sixty-five or seventy.

The two surgeries are usually done simultaneously, with removal of the ovaries performed routinely as "part of the hysterectomy" when, in fact, the ovary removal is almost always entirely unnecessary. In many cases it is done as a prophylactic measure; the organs are removed "while the surgeon is in there anyway," before they become diseased.

Some women who have had hysterectomies do not know whether they have had their ovaries removed. Others agreed to the removal without really knowing what they were agreeing to, or without realizing that hysterectomy itself is an *elective* procedure. Few, if any, know anything at all about the disadvantages of such surgery.

That's the sort of thing that happened to Miranda J.

When I was twenty-two I got a pain in my abdomen. I went to the hospital. They told me they had to do an exploratory operation and shot me full of morphine. When I came to, my uterus and ovaries were gone.

I cried and screamed because I was so upset. I had wanted children. I asked them how they could do a thing like that to me. They said I had an infection, that before I went into surgery I had signed a paper saying anything they did was all right. I have no memory of signing anything.

Sex hasn't meant anything to me since that operation, although I really loved it before. The doctors told me to wait until I was in my late thirties when I would be at my prime. I'm thirty-seven now and still waiting. I haven't recovered my sex drive. When I ask them about it, they just shrug and say I'm very unusual.

The United States has twice the hysterectomy rate of England and Sweden. Doctors' wives have more hysterectomies proportionately than any other group. Black women have twice as many hysterectomies as white women, although poor white women are not exempt from hysterectomy being used as a form of sterilization abuse.

Countless welfare mothers have been given vaginal hysterectomies, which leave no abdominal scars, without their previous knowledge or consent. The medical profession terms this sort of surgery a Mississippi Appendectomy.

Hysterectomy rates, which vary substantially in different regions of the United States, are lowest in the west. The northeast is next in frequency, then the north central section of the country. The rate is highest in the south.

Total hysterectomies have been performed since the mid-1940s. Prior to that time, gynecologists and surgeons performed what were called "subtotal hysterectomies," a procedure which left a cervical stump. Subtotals were faster; the patient didn't have the opportunity to bleed as much as during a total hysterectomy. In those days there was usually a lack of adequate blood for transfusions.

In some cases the retained cervix became cancerous, although it is entirely possible that those women would have gotten cancer anyway. With the advent of improved surgical techniques and supporting technologies, total hysterectomy became the surgery of doctors' choice. Legal and social changes in the late 1960s, particularly the emphasis on limiting population (abortion was illegal), brought about increased acceptance of sterilization as a means of contraception. For the first time, gynecologists recommended that hospitals no longer require a medical staff committee to review requests for sterilization based on parity and age.

Dr. Ralph Wright, a Connecticut gynecologist and an outspoken advocate of hysterectomy, attempted to explain why tissue committees were being presented with such large numbers of manifestly healthy uteruses. Widely quoted in obstetrics and gynecology journals, he wrote and spoke of "radical changes" in indications for hysterectomy.

Concerning sterilization he wrote: "To sterilize a patient and allow her to keep a useless and potentially lethal organ is incompatible with modern gynecologic concepts. Hysterectomy is the only logical approach to surgical sterilization."

This was the same physician who wrote, regarding cancer prevention, ". . . when the patient has completed her family, total hysterectomy should be performed as a prophylactic procedure. Under these circumstances, the uterus becomes a useless, bleeding, symptom-producing, potentially cancer-bearing organ and, therefore, should be removed."

In response to Wright's mind-boggling pronouncement, Dr. Stanley Friedman replied: "From 1960 to 1965 the death rate from prostatic cancer was about equal to that from all uterine cancers (National Vital Statistics Division and Bureau of the Census, United States). Applying Wright's logic of 'one basic principle,' it would seem equally rational to perform elective prostatectomy on every male whose wife is to undergo elective hysterectomy."

However, many physicians agreed with Dr. Wright's thinking, and still do. In his book, *A Woman Talks with Her Doctor: A Comprehensive Guide to Women's Health Care,* Dr. Charles E. Flowers, Jr., says: "Many women resist a hysterectomy because they associate the loss of their uterus with the loss of their femininity. I am fully aware that the loss of reproductivity can be threatening to many women, but the argument that the uterus is an essential aspect of femininity is simply not true. The uterus has one signal purpose: to carry and nourish the growing fetus. The uterus has no relationship whatsoever to a woman's sexuality or her ability to make love . . . sometimes the ovaries are removed because they are diseased or cancerous or the woman has endometriosis. Other times the ovaries are removed in conjunction with a hysterectomy as a preventive measure. However, if a woman is already menopausal, if she has already stopped menstruating, and she is having a hysterectomy for fibroids or some other condition, I believe her ovaries should be removed at the same time so they won't later become a source of ovarian cancer . . . if the woman's sex life was good before the operation, it's going to continue to be good. Just because she can no longer ovulate or conceive does not mean she cannot enjoy sex and have a good strong orgasm."

Whether or not gynecologists agreed with either rationale, physicians attending a general meeting of the American College of Obstetricians and Gynecologists on June 15, 1971, voted by applause to support sterilization as an appropriate medical indication for hysterectomy.

Sterilization then became a primary indication for hysterectomy. Men whose religions forbade birth control or abortion welcomed it, as did their wives—at least until after the surgery was done.

Many men still think hysterectomy means open sesame for sex. Women report that after their surgeries they are approached in a sexual way by male business and social associates. The woman has been "cleaned out" so she's safe for sex. They don't have to worry about getting her pregnant.

A whopping 68.5 percent of the vaginal hysterectomies performed at the University Hospital and Wayne County General Hospital in Ann Arbor, Michigan, between 1965 and 1970 were sterilizations for "socioeconomic" and "multiparity" reasons.

In 1970, 20 to 25 percent of hysterectomies done at Los Angeles County University of Southern California Medical Center were solely or primarily for sterilization.

The rate of sterilization by hysterectomy rose 293 percent between June 1968 and January 1970. California Blue Cross reported an increase of 79 percent in hysterectomies during just the first six months of 1970. Of 242 selected hysterectomies performed at the time of cesarean sections at the University of Arkansas Medical Center between 1970 and 1974, 68 percent were for sterilization.

The total number of hysterectomies performed nationally, as reported by NCHS, rose from 525,000 in 1970 to 690,000 in 1973, an increase of more than 30 percent.

Were women developing a plague of pelvic disease across

the country? No, only a plague of doctors. Shockingly, numerous findings prove that changes in hysterectomy rates vary in ways that correlate directly with the number of surgeons in a given area or the number of hospital beds available.

Retrospective reviews of hospital charts have repeatedly revealed that at least 30 percent of that bloody harvest was *not* medically justified; sterilization or so-called "cancer prevention" were the reasons.

In 1976 Blue Cross-Blue Shield advised subscribers to get a second and third opinion before agreeing to any elective surgery. The recommendation was based in part on various medical audits that showed that in many regions of the United States more than 40 percent of the hysterectomies and oophorectomies involved removal of normal organs.

In 1977 the hazards of indiscriminate surgery prompted a Congressional investigation. Predictably, the principal spokesman for the American Medical Association rose to the surgeons' defense. Dr. James H. Sammons, executive vice-president of the AMA, said the increase in hysterectomies was due to their elective use as a "convenient form of sterilization and to their prophylactic use to eliminate the possibility of uterine cancer in future years." Dr. Sammons asserted that while the surgery could not be considered clinically necessary for either of these reasons, it was "beneficial to women with excessive anxiety and therefore necessary."

How many surgeons would cure a man's anxiety about developing cancer of the penis by cutting it off? It's almost too ridiculous to mention, but that's exactly what's been happening to thousands of American women.

Cancer prevention is considered by some physicians to be an indication for hysterectomy itself; cutting an organ out before it has a chance to become cancerous. Complete hysterectomy to "prevent" cancer is being done every day in surgeries across the country. But certain physicians in positions of national leadership are distressed at the concept of hysterectomies being performed for preventive reasons.

Dr. Franz Ingelfinger, distinguished gastroenterologist who

edited the prestigious *New England Journal of Medicine* from 1967 to 1977, declares: "Once a physician starts removing healthy tissue for fear of cancer, he's gone too far."

The most frequent reason women seek gynecological care is for periodic genital and breast examinations to detect cancer. PAP examinations can lead directly to hysterectomies by revealing an abnormal condition such as severe dysplasia (a form of endometriosis), carcinoma in situ (cancer of the uterus), or invasive carcinomas (cancers) of the cervix.

PAP examinations can also lead indirectly to hysterectomies. If, upon pelvic examination, the gynecologist finds an abnormal condition such as uterine myomas (tumor containing muscle tissue), mild cervical dysplasia (abnormal changes in cervix tissue), or minimal prolapse of the uterus without associated pain or pressure, he may recommend hysterectomy.

These conditions by themselves would not medically justify hysterectomy. The woman can easily be "sold" hysterectomy with the argument that the uterus will probably develop more disease in time so it would be a good idea to remove it before that happens.

Some surgeons recommend the procedure to alleviate what they call "the drudgery of the menses," and still others because it is beneficial to the physician himself. "It decreases the frequency of unpleasant, humiliating pelvic exams and allows better utilization of health personnel, facilities and time."

Removal of normal ovaries at the time of hysterectomy is a common procedure. It is felt by the medical profession that such removal saves the .01 percent of women who otherwise might die from ovarian cancer. (This is also assuming that hormonal replacement therapy does not increase the chance of developing a malignancy of any remaining organ such as the breasts or the liver.)

Removal of the ovaries is comparatively simple when done at the time of uterus removal. Some doctors say they might as well be removed when the uterus is taken out because they'll very likely be severely damaged by the surgical procedure itself.

Dr. David R. Reuben, in his book, *How to Get More Out of Sex,* claims: "Hysterectomy doesn't have to be the end of sex for a woman. Like the old hospital joke, hysterectomy only takes out the baby carriage—it leaves the playpen intact. Most hysterectomies, even if the ovaries are not actually removed, bring on a 'surgical menopause.' Since the ovaries are such delicate structures, the cutting and crushing that goes on generally puts them essentially out of business."

Women who have a history of cancer in their families may decide to have their ovaries removed at the time of hysterectomy as a preventive measure. But it must be pointed out that the metabolic and endoctrine disturbances that develop when oophorectomy is performed are not reversed by the customary estrogen replacement. Even a small increase in the frequency of atherosclerotic heart disease, which frequently results from the loss of ovarian and uterine function, could offset any potential gain from cancer prevention.

In discussing cancer prevention surgery, researchers assume that a woman freed of the risk of one type of cancer would not be subject to a disproportionately higher risk of death from another cause, such as heart failure. Also, hysterectomy is not always the preferred treatment of uterine cancers. It would seem that the benefits of prophylactic surgery have been greatly overestimated. There is less chance that a woman will die from uterine cancer than that she will die when a hysterectomy is performed.

What are the health risks of hysterectomy?

Death is, of course, always a concern when any major surgery is undertaken for purely elective reasons. Although the mortality *rate* is low, the number of hysterectomies performed each year is so large that the resultant number of deaths is substantial. Each year more than six hundred women die as a result of complications from hysterectomy. How many die later from what may be certainly called residual effects, no one knows. The reported mortality rate for abdominal hysterectomy is .17 percent and for vaginal hysterectomy, .08 percent. These figures do not include women who died with pelvic malignancies.

Operative and postoperative complications are common with this type of surgery. These operative complications include bleeding as well as bladder, urethral, and rectal injuries suffered during surgery. If severe, such bleeding requires transfusions. The other complications require corrective surgery either at the time of the operation or following surgery, if the damage is not discovered when it is done.

Winifred F., a forty-year-old mother of three, said that she suffered pain, discharge, and a general feeling of total exhaustion for weeks following her hysterectomy, which was done because she was having discomfort with her periods. Her doctor told her it would be best to have "all that stuff taken out." She said she felt like she had an abcessed tooth at the top of her vaginal canal. When her fever shot to 104, she was rushed to the hospital, opened up again, and a large abscess was found.

"I'm terribly angry at myself for allowing the surgery," Winifred says now. "I would have been much better off if I'd just walked out of that doctor's office."

Fever is the most common postoperative complication but hemorrhage and transfusion, urinary dysfunction, wound and pelvic infections, intestinal obstruction, and thromboembolic disease are far too frequent, according to researchers now studying the problem.

In a Stanford study, 7.5 percent of nonemergency abdominal hysterectomy patients experienced moderate to life-threatening complications. The study showed there was some degree of morbidity in 64 percent of the nonemergency abdominal hysterectomy patients seven days after surgery.

In another study involving six hundred patients, 5 percent had a second operation—eight during the initial hospital stay, twenty-two returning to the hospital later. The second operations were for incisional hernias, intestinal obstruction, vaginal hemorrhage, intra-abdominal hemorrhage, septic vaginal or pelvic hematomas, stress incontinence, ovarian cysts, appendicitis, prolapsed Fallopian tubes, and ulcer in the sacral region.

There is little documentation on how rapidly hysterectomy patients recover their normal functional level. The sparse studies that exist indicate that hysterectomy patients report an average of 11.9 months to recover fully from surgery. This compares with a three-month recovery period for cholecystectomy (gall bladder removal), appendectomy, or partial mastectomy patients.

Depression is a particularly common psychological disturbance following hysterectomy. A survey conducted in England showed that depression, both treated with antidepressive drugs and untreated, was suffered by 70 percent of the women who had undergone such surgery, compared to only 30 percent of women who had undergone different kinds of surgeries.

A significant increase in visits to physicians for "neuroses and psychiatric disorders" was reported in a study from Manitoba. Researchers say that most of this increase was accounted for by women in the 20- to 39-year-old age group, particularly those who underwent removal of the ovaries.

One researcher in the United States found that 7 percent of 729 women who had undergone hysterectomy were referred to psychiatrists within a period of four and one-half years after their surgeries. This referral rate was two and one-half times the rate expected for a matched group of women in the general population. Of these psychiatric referrals, 80 percent occurred within the first two years following hysterectomy. Women undergoing hysterectomy in the absence of severe pelvic disease such as cancer were referred for psychiatric care twice as often as those who had severe pelvic disease.

A list of medically appropriate indications for hysterectomy was issued by the Professional Standards Review Organizations (PSRO) in 1977. Included were malignant and premalignant disease of the endometrium (mucus membrane of the uterus) and cervix; fibroma (tumor) of the cervix, fundus, or broad ligament; abnormal bleeding; and prolapsed uterus (protrusion of the uterus through the vaginal orifice). If the parts were close to malignant or infectious disease—such as cancer of the colon or tubal infections—or the conditions were in conjunction with vaginal repair, hysterectomy was also medically justified. Excluded from the list was sterilization in the absence of ongoing uterine disease.

Intended to include all acceptable medical indications for hysterectomy from saving life at one end to simply improving it at the other, these indications did not alone dictate hysterectomy as the only, or even the best, means of treatment.

The Executive Board of the American College of Obstetricians and Gynecologists distinguished five levels of urgency for hysterectomy: emergency, mandatory, urgent, advisable, and elective.

Examples of the five levels are: An emergency would be intra-abdominal hemorrhaging, such as that caused by a ruptured ecotopic pregnancy. The presence of a malignancy like an adenocarcinoma of the endometrium would call for mandatory surgery. Abnormal uterine bleeding requiring further diagnostic evaluation or definitive treatment is urgent. The advisable level is characterized by a condition like pelvic relaxation, such as that associated with urinary stress incontinence. Elective surgical procedures are those such as sterilization for family planning purposes. Elective hysterectomies would also include those for prophylaxis against potential disease such as uterine cancer.

The PSRO medical indications for hysterectomy specifically state that sterilization by vaginal or abdominal hysterectomy is acceptable only in the presence of concomitant uterine disease. The Medicare law specifically excludes reimbursement of hysterectomy for sterilization.

Some physicians consider hysterectomy the treatment of choice for economically disadvantaged women because such women have a greater risk of malignancy and are less likely to seek medical care. They cannot afford it. Socioeconomically disadvantaged women are at the highest risk of developing cervical cancer. For reasons as yet unknown they are not as likely to develop endometrial cancer, however, as endometrial cancer primarily affects middle and upper income women.

To lessen the abuse of this crippling surgery for minor benefits to the patients and major economic benefits for the physician, some medical experts feel that the elective hysterectomy policy should be directed toward implementation of the standards of care as developed by the PSRO program and the reimbursement policy of the Department of Health and Human Services.

This is unlikely to become a reality, however. Small successes have been achieved in limiting the numbers of elective hysterectomies by medical audit and peer review in certain individual institutions. But attempting to audit hysterectomies on a continual basis at the national level would be a formidable task. Under the present conditions of reimbursement incentives, such an attempt could not succeed. To disapprove indications for hysterectomy such as sterilization would only encourage further misrepresentation of the diagnosis.

The written medical records are not reliable. In many cases the true indications for surgery are not included in a patient's hospital chart for reasons including peer review; nonreimbursement; and patient, physician, or hospital religious affiliations that make it expedient to write in only approved reasons for hysterectomy such as "abnormal bleeding" and "prolapsed uterus." Although these two indications are consistent with a pathology report of "normal uterus," they *would* pass inspection faster than "back problem," which some surgeons give as indication for hysterectomy.

Indications for hysterectomies on hospital charts change to reflect the times. Now, more and more "prolapsed uteruses" are noted, the increase apparently due to changes in hospital practice to accommodate elective hysterectomy for sterilization if third-party payments for hysterectomies for sterilization are unpredictable.

Sometimes the decision for surgery is made primarily by the doctor, sometimes by the patient. Sometimes a woman thinks she herself has made the decision when, in fact, she has been subtly influenced by the doctor's sales pitch. Many women, after talking with their physicians, choose hysterectomy to avoid "messy" menstruation, to ensure a safe birth control method, or from a fear of future cancer.

Numerous findings indicate that changes in hysterectomy rates are not a function of changes in pelvic disease or age patterns among women. Hysterectomy rates have been shown to correlate with the ratio of surgeon to patient and the availability of hospital beds. Also, when medical audits are enforced, the hysterectomy rates have dropped sharply.

A lot of hysterectomy involves salesmanship on the part of physicians. Unfortunately, it's all too easy for a woman to believe, consciously or subconsciously, that an organ she cannot see, that bleeds regularly, will eventually become cancerous—especially if her doctor skillfully hints at this possibility.

Yet one patriarchal family doctor once said: "If women were not meant to have these parts after production of their families, nature would have arranged for them to dry up around age forty-five."

Chapter Two

CURRENT MEDICAL
REASONS FOR
HYSTERECTOMY

About once every thirty seconds a woman in the United States follows her physician's advice to undergo a hysterectomy, a potentially dangerous and fairly expensive surgery costing approximately $4,710.

What exactly is a hysterectomy? It is the surgical removal of the entire uterus (or womb) and only the uterus. The uterus itself includes the fundus (upper third), the body of the uterus (middle third) and the cervix of the uterus (lower third). The terms total hysterectomy, complete hysterectomy, and pan hysterectomy mean exactly the same thing—removal of the uterus in its entirety. If the Fallopian tubes and ovaries are also removed, as they are in approximately half of all hysterectomies, that additional portion of the operation is called a salpingo-oophorectomy.

Hysterectomies are usually done to correct or alleviate one of the following conditions: uterine bleeding, fibroid tumors, pelvic inflammatory disease, chronic pelvic pain, prolapse of the uterus, cancer, obstetrical catastrophe.

The surgical removal of the uterus is accomplished either through the vagina or through an incision in the wall of the abdomen. The method usually depends on the medical reason for the operation or the disinclination of the patient to have a scar. If a woman has a prolapsed (dropped) uterus and cystocele (drooping bladder, usually caused by multiple childbirths), most doctors will perform a vaginal hysterectomy which allows easy access to the uterus and enables the gynecologist to resuspend the bladder in its normal position. There are physicians who believe that if a woman has borne even one child, she needs a bladder tuck.

A woman with large bulky fibroid tumors of the uterus is generally a candidate for abdominal hysterectomy. Also, the presence of scar tissue or adhesions from pelvic infections, inflammation, or endometriosis (uterine tissue growing in the abdomen outside the uterus), would also make abdominal hysterectomy the surgery of medical choice, as would the necessity to remove an ovarian tumor along with the uterus. Most surgeons prefer the abdominal approach which allows them to look at the ovaries and tubes for possible removal at the time of hysterectomy. Removal of the ovaries is usually a judgment made by the surgeon at the time of surgery.

Uterine bleeding is frequently one of the symptoms of a condition called adenomatous hyperplasia, an endometrial condition in which the lining of the uterus becomes hyperactive because of a hormonal imbalance. Clinically, this condition can be considered mild, moderate, or severe. If the condition advances to the severe stage it can, over a period of time, become what is called atypical adenomatous hyperplasia, which is the same as early carcinoma in situ of the endometrium. Many doctors say that if a patient is in her forties and the pathology reports indicate that she has mild to moderate adenomatous hyperplasia, she can be successfully treated with synthetic progesterones, taken either orally or by intramuscular injections. Over a period of time, such hormone therapy will result in a more normal endometrium.

Many doctors, on the other hand, would strongly recommend hysterectomy, including removal of the tubes and ovaries, whether the condition was mild, moderate, or severe.

Endometriosis has been called a closet disease; few women have wanted to know what it is and even fewer have wanted to talk about it. It has been called a "career woman's disease, because if you have children early and frequently, you won't have the disease." The reality might be that the disease is diagnosed more in educated, assertive women because it takes a persistent, educated woman to get a diagnosis, according to Mary Lou Ballweg, co-founder of the Endometriosis Association. It *is* a baffling condition in which tissue lining the uterus appears outside the uterine cavity. This webby tissue can also be found on the ovaries, on the peritoneum (the layer of tissue that coats the abdominal cavity and internal organ surfaces), and on the interior walls of the pelvic cavity. The cause is unknown and symptoms differ, but most women have pain as a symptom—pain that is in some cases at a level greater than the pain of labor.

Treatment for endometriosis has ranged from hormonal therapy to conservative surgery in which growths are removed, to hysterectomy and removal of the ovaries.

Thousands of hysterectomies are done for fibroid tumors, which are solid growths of muscle tissue and fibrous connective tissue that are found in the uterine wall. Fibroids, also known as myomas or leiomyomas, can be as tiny as a pea or as large as a full-term unborn child. Fibroids are nearly always benign.

The amount of pain and discomfort fibroids cause depends on their location and the size and stage of growth. Symptoms of fibroids can range from nothing at all to heavy bleeding, longer periods, passing of clots, and a feeling of heaviness or pressure and lower abdominal pain not connected with menstruation. If large fibroids grow on the back wall of the uterus, they can cause painful intercourse, low back pain, and leg cramps. If they grow on the front wall, they can put pressure on the bladder and cause frequent urination. Other symptoms can include dizziness and possibly fainting if bleeding has been severe. Many women have these symptoms and don't know they have fibroids until a doctor detects them during a pelvic examination.

Lucy N., thirty-five, had three children—a boy of twelve, and a girl ten from her first marriage, and a small son, a year and a half, by her present husband. She wanted one more child, someone to grow up with the youngest.

During a routine pelvic exam, Lucy's gynecologist informed her that her uterus was covered with small fibroids. Immediately Lucy was panic-stricken. She had several friends who had undergone hysterectomies because of fibroids. She knew she must have an operation—fast.

Lucy's gynecologist reassured her. "You don't need a hysterectomy. These things come and go. I'll keep my eye on them. If you start growing one the size of a basketball, then we'll get serious."

Lucy wasn't satisfied. She was afraid *not* to have a hysterectomy. She consulted three other doctors, all of whom strongly advised hysterectomy at once.

"I almost had the operation," she said. "I talked it over with my husband. We both had a lot of confidence in my regular gynecologist so we decided to abide by his decision. And am I glad we did! I had my fourth child, a daughter. The fibroids went away. My friends with their hysterectomies are having all sorts of problems while I feel like a million dollars. That gynecologist of mine—I revere him! All women should be so lucky!"

Lucy is not unusual. Too often women are naive about hysterectomy and plead for the surgery. If they're lucky, they will have a doctor who talks them out of it. If they're unlucky, they'll shop around until they find one only too happy to operate.

Many doctors, however, concur that fibroids constitute a reason for hysterectomy. Dr. Sheldon H. Cherry, writing in *For Women of All Ages, a Gynecologist's Guide to Modern Female Health Care,* says: "In the older woman or in the young woman with fibroids who has completed her family, a hysterectomy is the normal procedure. This eliminates the possibility of developing more fibroids and also prevents future uterine malignancy."

While a number of doctors recommend hysterectomy for nearly any type of fibroid tumor, especially if the woman has had her family, doesn't desire children, or is forty or over, others don't operate unless the fibroids cause infertility, pain, prolonged or heavy bleeding during the menstrual period, or if they have grown so large they are pressing on the bladder or the Fallopian tubes.

Chronic and recurrent pelvic inflammatory disease, in which the tubes and ovaries are nearly destroyed by both previous and recurring infection, is usually treated by hysterectomy as is chronic pelvic pain. Chronic pain can be caused by a wide variety of troubles, ranging from scar tissue to a kind of undiagnosed pain, where nothing is actually found to be wrong but the patient seems to benefit mentally by having her organs removed.

Another common medical indication for hysterectomy is prolapse of the uterus. While some cases *are* severe, many are mild or insignificant. One doctor said: "Lots of hospitals have a lot of surgical cases of partial prolapse of the uterus. In the trade, it's called Catholic sterilization. The beauty of a prolapse is that you don't have to have much of a pathology. Who can prove, after the fact of surgery, that a woman's uterus was sagging a bit?"

Although the alternative to hysterectomy for sterilization of a woman is tubal ligation, patients are usually urged to have a hysterectomy. The two reasons commonly given by the medical profession for preferring hysterectomy over tubal ligation are that hysterectomy is 100 percent effective in preventing conception and it removes the chance of future uterine/cervical disease.

Obstetrical catastrophies such as uterine rupture, another indication for hysterectomy, are extremely rare.

While uterine cancer is usually an indication for surgery, hysterectomy can be avoided in some cases by treating early cancer of the cervix. The majority of women with this condition are under thirty; most are concerned with their ability to bear children, so alternative treatments are becoming commonplace. A so-called cone biopsy of the cervix can be definitive treatment for very early cervical cancer. Cryosurgery (freezing) and the use of laser beam to destroy involved tissue are extensively used.

Ovarian cancer, formerly thought to be one of the most deadly of cancers, needn't be nearly so deadly if the right kind of attention is paid to its early warning signs and if the best available therapies are routinely applied. At present, however, early symptoms of ovarian cancer are usually ignored or dismissed as insignificant, and proper diagnosis is not made until the cancer is in a relatively advanced stage.

If ovarian cancer has afflicted more than one of a woman's close blood relatives, statistics tell us that she is more likely than other women to develop the disease herself. Such a woman should have herself watched closely for possible signs of the disease. In some cases, women with long family histories of this cancer are concerned enough to choose to have their ovaries removed while the organs are still healthy; before doing so, however, they should study the other problems that ovarian removal can cause.

According to Dr. Vincent T. DeVita, Jr., director of the National Cancer Institute in Bethesda, Maryland, "Ovarian cancer tends to be undertreated because it is understaged." Dr. DeVita explains that the surgery performed as the first line of treatment often does not go far enough to detect the presence of cancer in other tissues. As a result, surgeons may not realize that the disease has already spread and, thus, may fail to suggest further treatments for their patients. Jane E. Brody, writing in *The New York Times,* emphasizes that it is very important for the surgeon who operates on a woman with ovarian cancer to be extremely familiar with the disease as well as with all the abdominal sites to which it is inclined to spread. She recommends that within the limits imposed by the woman's presurgical health, the operation should be as extensive as possible, including the removal of tissues such as the omentum (a fatty pad that hangs down from the large intestine) and the sampling of cells from the diaphragm and other tissues for careful microscopic examination.

It has long been thought by the medical profession that ovarian cancer in its early stages produces no symptoms. But, according to Dr. Hugh R. K. Barber, a gynecologist at Lenox Hill Hospital in New York and a recognized expert on this disease, many victims, when carefully questioned, *report having had gastrointestinal symptoms that were ignored or dismissed as unimportant for months before their cancers were diagnosed.* He urges all middle-aged and older women who develop symptoms of indigestion—gas, a feeling of fullness after eating small amounts of food, belching, or heartburn—to have themselves checked promptly and, if no cause is found, to be examined by a gynecologist for possible ovarian cancer.

Ovarian cancer is primarily a disease of older women. The risk starts rising at age forty and peaks at seventy-seven, with most cases being diagnosed among women in their sixties. Although the precise cause or causes of ovarian cancer have not been determined, recent studies have identified factors that may play a role in promoting or preventing its development.

Women who bear their first child before the age of twenty-two or who have lots of children are less likely than others to develop ovarian cancer. It is not known whether it is the age at which the first child is born or the number of children a woman has that is the protective factor.

Another group of women who warrant closer examination are those who, two or more years after completing menopause, are found to have ovaries as large as those in premenopausal women. Dr. Barber says that "a so-called normal-sized ovary in a postmenopausal woman is abnormal," adding that any postmenopausal woman who starts bleeding vaginally should be immediately checked for the possibility of cancer.

Regarding the other common indications for hysterectomy such as abnormal uterine bleeding or flooding periods, severe infection, fibroids, prolapse of the uterus, certain medical experts assert that all can be treated medically—not surgically.

If a woman wants to keep her uterus, but truly does need surgery for troublesome fibroids, she should consider having a myomectomy, an operation in which only the fibroids are removed; the uterus is left intact. It may be difficult to find a doctor who performs myomectomies. In 1983 there were 37,000 myomectomies performed compared to 672,000 hysterectomies, approximately half of which were due to fibroids. If a woman's own gynecologist has no experience with myomectomies, she should look for a doctor affiliated with a teaching hospital or with a major medical center.

Often a woman with fibroids has difficulty conceiving if the fibroid tumors block the Fallopian tubes. A myomectomy would correct this condition without sacrificing the woman's uterus.

About 90 percent of women who are infertile because of fibroids can become pregnant after having myomectomies. The few physicians who perform these procedures recommend attempting pregnancy as soon as possible after the six-month waiting period following surgery.

Regarding the removal of a woman's ovaries, most gynecologists feel that if the patient is in her late thirties or early forties, if her menstrual periods are irregular or if she's starting to have hot flashes and is in what is called a prodromal menopausal state (just before the menses stops), she should undergo hysterectomy together with removal of her tubes and ovaries.

Physicians believe that at this point in a woman's life her ovaries are beginning to atrophy, that they're not going to be producing hormones much longer and they should come out. In short, they feel that ovaries have a limited usefulness.

But the anecdotal evidence gathered for this book indicates that women who had their uteruses removed but who retained even a piece of an ovary did not suffer many of the painful changes undergone by women who had lost all of their ovaries.

It would seem from certain scholarly studies that an atrophic ovary, or even a shred of an ovary, does serve a necessary feminine function.

Chapter Three

WHAT WOMEN DON'T KNOW <u>CAN</u> HURT THEM

Second to the scandal of hysterectomy itself, the most horrible deception practiced on women has been the medical profession's assurance that the surgery will have no adverse effect on other bodily functions or on their sexual desire.

Said one kindly physician who has been treating women for three decades: "Why should I mention sexual dysfunction to a woman facing hysterectomy? She has enough problems. Of course sexual dysfunction occurs. It is one of the most common yet least talked about results of a hysterectomy that includes removal of both ovaries."

Other physicians categorically deny that such dysfunction can occur as a result of hysterectomy, claiming any reports to that effect are nothing more than old wives' tales, passed down from older generations in an effort to alarm younger women. Others say that if such apparent postsurgical effects do occur, the reasons are entirely psychological, never physical.

Many doctors smile at the sense of loss some women express when faced with hysterectomy. "My dear, they're only your reproductive organs," they console. "You won't even know they're gone."

A woman's reproductive organs occupy at least one-third of her inner abdominal space. More importantly, they represent a vital part of her womanhood. Medical science has not as yet explored the aftereffects of such surgery. Our present system of medical care gives little or no thought to how a woman *feels*—mentally, emotionally, physically—following hysterectomy.

There are women who have no forebodings prior to surgery and suffer no sexual dysfunction later but *do* suffer an unexpected emotional toll. These women find that the matter-of-fact explanations given by their physicians in no way prepare them for the ensuing psychological stress. Significantly, many of these women never connect that emotional problem or stress to their operations. Some go to therapists for entirely different reasons. The revelation comes when the therapist identifies the problem as a direct result of the hysterectomy.

Deep down, these women are troubled with what troubles most women in this situation. An era in their lives has ended. Whether or not they wanted more children—or *any* children—that option is now closed. Physical motherhood has become an impossibility. An integral part of who they are has been lost. For most women, hysterectomy is an emotionally devastating time.

Others suffer both psychological and sexual loss. Unfortunately, there is far more substance to women's fear of hysterectomy than has been credited. Anaphrodisia, a dulling of sexual appetite, is a specific ailment involving altered hormonal balances, not a vague dreamy fear of advancing age, empty nests, and loss of youthful attractiveness.

To most women, the uterus is a highly significant organ. Its loss threatens their sexuality, their perception of themselves as females. We are all, male and female, sexual beings. We hope to be sexually desirable to others. Sexual desirability is a measure of worth among humans, as it is in the animal kingdom, where it is expressed in seasons of estrus and rut.

Nowadays, many women do not start their families until their late thirties or early to mid-forties, at an age that, in the past, most women were considered old. Lots of women today reach the peak of physical attractiveness in their late forties and fifties. This is a time of ripeness, of fulfillment, of savoring one's victories and understanding one's losses. It should be the best time of all for sex. How tragic that so many women have been surgically altered so that some of this pleasure is impossible!

In studies noting the adverse effects of hysterectomy, Dr. Niles Newton, behavioral psychologist and professor of psychiatry at Northwestern Medical School, explored what she terms "another consequence of hysterectomy, one that may not be important to male gynecologists but certainly is of extreme importance to their patients—the suppression of libido following the surgery."

In her research, Dr. Newton found frightening results. She discovered reduced sexual drive in 60 percent of women who had had their uterus and both ovaries removed. Forty percent of the women who'd had hysterectomies never resumed sexual intercourse. Other researchers are finding that from 20 to 42 percent of women they study abstain from sexual intercourse following hysterectomy.

Yet, in the face of complaints from patients and of research such as Dr. Newton's, most doctors still deny this sequela of hysterectomy. For example, Dr. Harry C. Huneycutt writes in his book *All About Hysterectomy:* "Women who claim their interest in sex has vanished after hysterectomy are subsequently proven by psychologists to have disliked their husbands for years . . . the only physical tie-in I have seen for a woman's not enjoying sex as much is in that rare woman who enjoys the deep, jolting sensation when her partner's penis jars the uterus. For most women, this is a painful sensation, and they choose positions to avoid this feeling if their partners tend to penetrate that deeply."

Dr. Michael Carrera, author of *Sex: The Facts, The Acts & Your Feelings,* states: "Sexual interest and drive, and the ability to have orgasm, are not affected by hysterectomy . . . ovariectomy (or oophorectomy), the removal of both ovaries, is also called female castration . . . ovariectomy does not interfere with interest in, or enjoyment of, sex."

Dr. Bruce D. Shephard, writing with Carroll A. Shephard, R.N., Ph.D., in *The Complete Guide to Women's Health,* says: "There is no evidence that hysterectomy, with or without removal of the ovaries, alters sexual desire, responsiveness or satisfaction."

And Dr. W. Gifford-Jones says in his book *On Being a Woman:* "One of the most frequent old wives' tales concerns the operation causing some change in sexual function.

"What are the real facts about sex and its relationship to hysterectomy? The enjoyment of the sexual act is a mental phenomenon and is in no way dependent on whether the uterus or ovaries are present. One cannot change a person's attitude toward sex merely by removing an organ which has to do only with pregnancy and has nothing to do with sex. But of course the woman who has never enjoyed sex, or who has fallen out of love with her husband, finds her hysterectomy represents an excellent excuse for pushing her husband away. And undoubtedly she will find friends to support her stand. It is this type of woman who helps give the operation an unjustly bad reputation."

Doctors who blame the marriage for posthysterectomy sexual dysfunction have caused untold heartaches. Many women revealed during research that if they had been told that sexual dysfunction *could* occur, they and their mates would have been far more competent to cope with the resultant problems. Such is the story of Cindy W., whose doctor recommended a complete hysterectomy after the birth of her third child when Cindy was twenty-three.

The doctor had found some fibroid tumors in the walls of her uterus. Because Cindy and her husband, Jack, didn't want any more children, they weren't upset about the idea of an operation. Cindy's doctor told her he would take her ovaries, too, as it was so easy for them to become cancerous. He said she'd never know they were gone.

The operation was successful. On the second day Cindy was walking a bit and after a week she went home. Six weeks later a friend kept the children and Cindy and Jack went to bed early, taking the phone off the hook and pulling the blinds around the house.

"Nothing's going to spoil tonight," Jack said. "We've waited too long to be together again."

They undressed eagerly and lay on the bed. "Don't turn the lamp off," he whispered. "I want to look at you."

"But I've got a scar, Jack. You don't want to look at *that*."

"Yeah, but it's a smiley scar. Look how it curves up like a big grin. It's saying, 'Come on, Jack, come on in.' "

She laughed delightedly.

As hard as she tried, and as desperately as she wanted Jack, she couldn't climax.

"Don't worry, sweets, it's just too soon. Let me help you."

Using his mouth, he brought her to what she said was a "sort of a climax." She really wasn't sure. "It was funny. There wasn't any feeling *inside*. It was like it was all on the outside."

After another three months, with no improvement in her reaction to sex with her husband, Cindy consulted Dr. Warren. She told him she couldn't reach a climax. Nor did she desire sex.

"That wouldn't have anything to do with your operation," the doctor replied.

"But I never had any trouble before the operation."

"Cindy, I'm going to prescribe more estrogen for you," Dr. Warren said, swiveling around in his chair and making a few scrawls on a prescription pad. "Take these and come back in six weeks."

In six weeks she was back in the doctor's office. Things were no better. She still couldn't climax the way she had before. The only way she could achieve satisfaction—and then only occasionally—was if her husband spent at least half an hour manipulating her clitoris orally or with his fingers. Even with the occasional climax, she felt unfulfilled. She also complained of breaking out in heavy suffocating sweats.

"That means you're getting too much estrogen," he told her. "Let's cut back again. We have to adjust the dosage for each individual." Then he looked up from his prescription pad. "You've got to realize that there's nothing about the surgery that would account for your unhappiness in bed. Are you and Jack getting along?"

"Of course we are. And we were looking forward to sex after the surgery because we knew we wouldn't have to worry about pregnancy anymore."

"That's the way it should be, and will be again. Keep the faith."

Before the surgery, Cindy said, she and her husband had made love every night except during her menstrual periods—many times more than once a night. She distinctly remembered the first night Jack didn't approach her. She thought he was sick. Then she feared he was simply tired of all the manipulatory work he had to do first. "I went into the bathroom and bawled my eyes out," she said. "Jack was dead to the world. He didn't even wake up."

When five days had passed without Jack touching her, Cindy made the first move. She kissed him lingeringly, thinking that if she simulated her old passion, that might do the trick. They made love for over two hours. She couldn't climax. She finally pushed him away and lay crying on the bed.

"What's wrong with you?" he asked.

When she sobbed that she didn't know, he said, "The only thing that's different is that you had that operation. I'm going to see your doctor tomorrow."

When he came home the next night Jack looked grim. "Give the kids their dinner and get them to bed. You and I have to talk."

Later they sat on the sofa. "Okay, Cindy, here's the way it is," Jack said. "Dr. Warren said that if we're having trouble in bed there's something wrong with our marriage."

"But nothing *is* wrong, Jack. You know that."

"You can't come anymore. I'd say that's pretty damned wrong."

"I can't help it, Jack. You know how I try."

"Dammit. I don't want a woman to *try*, for God's sake! I want a woman to come because she's enjoying me so much she can't stop herself."

He stared into the fire, then took her hand. "Dr. Warren suggested I leave you alone for a month. Maybe by then you'll get over this block or whatever it is."

"You mean you're not going to sleep with me for a whole month?"

"I'll bunk down in here. If I was in the same bed, I'd take you in my sleep. We've both got to work at this seriously, Cindy. We've got to get you over this."

Slowly the month went by. The more Cindy slept alone, the more unsure of herself she became.

One day she left the kids with a friend and drove out into the woods to find Jack. He and his crew were taking down timber. She heard them long before she saw them—the toot, toot, toot warning whistle of the Cat, the whine of chain saws, the thud of trees falling, the scream of the rigging as it pulled logs up from the canyon.

"I can't lose him," she thought desperately as she watched him direct the complicated and dangerous business of timber harvesting.

When he saw her standing by the pick-up, he signaled the crew to go on working and clambered over the downed trees to her side. "What's wrong? Something with the kids?"

"No, Jack, I just needed to talk to you." She took his hands. "I love you, Jack. Please try to understand. Whatever is wrong, it isn't because I don't love you."

"Yeah, well." He looked off into the distance. "I just don't understand how you can turn off like that."

I'm losing him, she thought with a sick feeling in her stomach.

"I've gotta get back to work." He waved and strode back up the hill.

When the enforced platonic month was over, Cindy determined to become an actress. *If I don't feel anything, I'll act as if the roof is coming off. It won't hurt me and it might help my marriage.*

She put on a sterling performance. Jack wasn't fooled. He wouldn't leave her alone until he had forced a clitoral climax.

63

"Feel that?" he asked, his hand vibrating over her body. "That's what I feel you doing inside when you come the way you used to. No matter how much you yell and scream, if I don't feel *that*, I know you haven't come."

After that, things deteriorated. Jack started coming home later and later. Within a few months he was drinking heavily. Soon he began picking fights with her, then slamming out for the rest of the night. Some of his old girl friends gave her knowing looks when she ran into them at the local grocery store. Then she heard from a "kind" friend that Jack was frequently seen in the company of a striking-looking girl who was the bookkeeper for an international timber company.

One year later Cindy and Jack were divorced. There were terribly humiliating scenes, still too painful for her to discuss, in which she tried to get Jack back. She moved to a city where she knew no one. Jack was generous in his payments to her and the children. She found a day-care center, took dental technician's training, and is now employed by an oral surgeon. Jack has remarried.

"I understand Jack and I still love him," Cindy said. "Our problem was that he just couldn't understand that I still wanted to love him. He thought I didn't anymore. The doctor told him it was my fault. I guess somehow it was."

Cindy is now twenty-seven years old. She says she has friends with the same problem. "There wasn't anything wrong with them, either, until their operations. Women should be told the truth about hysterectomy. It isn't fair. It just isn't fair."

There is a stirring throughout the country as women begin to voice their discontent with the Great Hysterectomy Myth. Recently, one of the nation's largest women's magazines printed for the first time that sex life after hysterectomy "is affected in some cases." The brief paragraph went on to say that 10 to 39 percent of women who have had the surgery report sexual problems, but watered the statement down by adding that this is partly ascribed to "psychological reactions from the loss of the ability to have children."

Some professionals are more outspoken. Eleanor Katz-

---

man, marriage counselor and sex therapist, reports that 98 percent of the patients in her clinic are women who have lost sexual desire following hysterectomy. "I believe that if women truly understood what they're facing with the removal of these organs they wouldn't jump into the operation quite so fast," she said. "They'll find alternative measures to the scalpel if at all possible. What women don't know about hysterectomy can hurt them irrevocably for the rest of their lives."

The Conspiracy of Silence

Women are marvelous creatures, constructed in mysterious and wonderful ways, each one an entire universe unto herself.

They are also gullible, possessed of a desperate need to *believe*. Many steadfastly believe manifest untruths, no matter how moldy the old saw. Women believe advertising, even though they know its purpose is to sell, and cheerfully spend billions of dollars on cosmetics, fashions, spas, and other beauty-enhancing devices. They also believe doctors because they have been sold the idea that whatever a doctor decrees is right, which makes it easy to understand why otherwise intelligent women believe Old Saw No. 3,467—that sex will be better after hysterectomy.

Where is the man who believes that sex will be better after his penis is removed?

When a woman discovers that she has been robbed of her ability to enjoy sex, she accepts Old Saw No. 3,468—that, somehow, it's all her fault.

She then joins the Great Conspiracy of Silence. What woman wants to admit that she doesn't enjoy sex anymore? Such an admission in contemporary society would be as self-condemnatory as publicly renouncing belief in God, deodorant, and the silicon chip.

It is a fact that hysterectomy produces more sexual complications—physiological as well as psychological—than any other surgical procedure. In many women it creates a drastic change in the desire for and the experience of sex.

Now that Americans are spending an estimated $400 billion a year on health care (a stunning figure that exceeds the annual growth in gross national product and is still growing), women continue to undergo this surgery with little or no thought for its long-term effect.

Margaret W., a twenty-eight-year-old professional woman, said: "My marriage is ruined! My doctor says sex should be better since my hysterectomy. But it isn't. I want my husband with my head but I can't want him with my body."

There are untold thousands of women throughout the country who belong to the Great Conspiracy of Silence. What do these women do? Some are women whose marriages have foundered on the shoals of divorce. There no longer seems any real reason to have a man around. Others stay married, leading lives of quiet frustration, faking it in bed, hoping their partners won't notice the difference. Some have husbands who seek sexual solace elsewhere. Others experiment sexually in a sad and desolate search for what they have lost. The lucky ones have supportive mates who try to help them through this time of bewilderment and depression.

No matter what their degree of sophistication, pre-hysterectomy women seem to fall into two distinct categories: those who consider hysterectomy "just an operation, a necessary one," because their doctors said so; and those who want answers to the following questions:

- Will I still want sex after hysterectomy?
- If so, will it be pleasurable for me?
- Will it be pleasurable for my partner?
- Will I still be able to have orgasms?
- Will they feel as good as before?
- What happens to all the space that's left?
- Will I be thought a fool if I ask these questions?

Far too often what women are *told* by their physicians has very little to do with what *is*. Following hysterectomy a sexually distressed woman is likely to hear:

- Sex is 90% between your ears. You must have expected a loss of libido, so it happened.
- You're approaching the middle years. You can't expect the drive you had when you were twenty. (If you reply that you had it just before the surgery, you are told: "Be patient. Give it time.")
- You and your husband are having problems, aren't you? It's a cop-out to blame the surgery.
- Maybe you didn't really like sex before. Now surgery gives you a good excuse to avoid it.
- You can have an orgasm now and then with clitoral stimulation. What are you complaining about?
- There *are* other things in life beside sex. Maybe now is the time to develop other interests. After all, you had an exciting sex life for, how many years was it?

It is not women's fault that they do not understand the effect hysterectomy will have upon their entire beings until after the fact of surgery. When they search for the bread of knowledge, they are fed the vinegar of half-truth or no-truth. They are blandly lied to by the very experts they have consulted to learn the truth about their bodies.

Much of the literature available sings the praises of hysterectomy as a "beneficial" surgical procedure. "Don't be hysterical over hysterectomy!" trills an expensively produced booklet widely distributed in gynecologists' offices throughout the United States. "That most unfortunate old wives' tale that hysterectomy makes you less of a woman is totally groundless." No doubt a clever play on words, but the woman facing the loss of her female organs is searching for something more substantial than advertising hyperbole.

"Another old wives' tale, the most destructive of all," the booklet purrs on, "is that the woman is psychologically, in some unknown way, less of a sexual being. Yet the reproductive system is quite separate from her sexual apparatus. Women who have had hysterectomies can look forward to an active, satisfying sexual life."

It then states that if a man loses his testicles he has an insurmountable problem, not only in impregnating women, but in performing sexually. "Not so with a woman," it asserts didactically. "Then why do so many women, even if they don't give voice to it, feel their sexual performance will be limited after hysterectomy?

"Obviously only psychiatry can do justice to such a question!" the booklet goes on sadly. "Why there was even a time when it was believed that cutting the hair would deprive one of strength. Though we now know *that* is ridiculous, there are many people who don't fully know that it is equally as silly to believe that removing the uterus and ovaries reduces female sexuality.

"In fact," the booklet crescendoes, "this operation can actually result in a woman being *more* of a woman!"

More of a woman? The scalpeled woman will be more of a woman, will be improved by having something cut out?

A guide to understanding hysterectomy, produced for distribution in west coast gynecologists' offices, asks: "Did you know that one out of every four women will have a hysterectomy? In fact, more hysterectomies are performed each year than any other type of major surgery.

"Fortunately," we are assured, "it is one of the safest major operations. Because a hysterectomy can relieve chronic pain and excessive bleeding, and even curtail life-threatening illness, the majority of women are usually happier and more comfortable after surgery."

The booklet advises that a "world of myths surrounds hysterectomy—that the loss of your uterus will make you gain weight, bring on early change of life, or make you sexually unattractive. Nothing could be further from the truth," it trumpets. "Because the sole function of the uterus is to provide a place for a baby to grow, having a hysterectomy means only that you will no longer have your period and that you cannot become pregnant. Hysterectomy is one of the safest major operations you can have, and has been shown to be extremely beneficial for the majority of women who have had one. This booklet is intended to help answer your questions, and to reassure you that life without your uterus can be just as good—or better—than ever!"

The booklet is filled with full-color drawings of a post-hysterectomy woman leaping about, apparently pain free, wiggling her toes in bed with a man, swimming, playing tennis, gardening, bicycling, running.

The strong implication is that if a woman can walk after her surgery, she can have a satisfying sex life. This theme runs through most of the literature.

Sexual desire and enjoyment cannot be equated with being able to play tennis. Sex is a physical activity, of course, but a woman's body could go through the physical motions of sex just as her arm could go through the physical motions of swinging a tennis racket. She doesn't expect her arm to have an orgasm. She hopes her body will.

Recently a woman wrote to a syndicated medical advice column: "About five years ago I had a hysterectomy and ever since then I haven't cared for sex anymore. My husband is very affectionate and this is putting a strain on our marriage. Is there a solution to this problem?"

The answer she received? "There is no physical reason that removal of your uterus and ovaries should affect sexual enjoyment in the slightest. The only purpose of the uterus is to receive a fertilized egg and nourish it after conception. It is not necessary for sexual pleasure. In fact, the uterus is anatomically pretty well removed from the scene of the 'action' so far as intercourse is concerned. So your problem would seem to be in your own mind or in the state of your marriage outside of sex. If you cannot work things out on this basis, see a marriage counselor, but don't lay it on your hysterectomy."

Was this woman helped? Not at all. She was given a strong push toward self-doubt and guilt and told that her problem is in her head or in the state of her marriage. It was certainly *not* the fault of her surgery. Never! Can anyone blame her husband for suspecting his wife of cooling toward him? Of course not. He has his wife's doctor to back up his suspicions.

Another recent medical column contained this question: "My doctor has taken everything out—my ovaries, my uterus, my cervix—so now would you please tell me if I can have an orgasm with sexual intercourse? This is bothering my mind very much." The answer was, "Yes, you can still have orgasms. The sensations of the vagina are intact."

If the woman cares to research this answer, she *will* have a problem. She has been told that the sensations of the vagina are intact and will carry her through to orgasm. But Masters and Johnson, the acclaimed sex research and therapy team, say that vaginal stimulation adds little, if anything, to the total arousal elicited by intercourse. According to them, sensory receptors are almost absent from the vaginal wall; they discount the role of sensations from the vagina in building up to orgasmic fulfillment.

Exponents of the G-spot, on the other hand, say there is a sensitive area just behind the front wall of the vagina between the back of the pubic bone and the cervix. Researchers named this area the Grafenberg spot, after Dr. Ernst Grafenberg, the first modern physician to describe it. The role of the G-spot is at present a controversial theory among sex researchers.

So the lady finds herself in a dilemma. The doctor tells her she's okay, she still has her vagina. Masters and Johnson say forget the vagina, there's not much feeling there anyway. Grafenberg supporters hail the G-spot as a source of intense pleasure. Others say there is no such thing.

What nobody considers, regardless of the experts and their arguments, is what's really at the heart of the issue: *how sex felt to this woman before her surgery and how it feels to her now.*

Some years ago Lauren R. fell in love with a much older man after being divorced from her first husband. She had one child from her marriage, a little boy, whom she adored.

About six months into her new relationship, a gynecologist confirmed Lauren's suspicion that she was pregnant. She happily informed her lover.

Rather than rejoicing with her, he sped back to his former wife, effected a reconciliation, and issued an ultimatum: Lauren was to immediately undergo an abortion. If she persisted in having the child, he and his wife (they had quickly remarried) would sue for custody of Lauren's baby and the wife would raise the baby as her own. In addition, the lover would give all the facts to Lauren's first husband, who would immediately sue for custody of Lauren's little boy.

This occurred when a vindictive ex-mate could cause an awful lot of problems for a woman who was pregnant outside of marriage. Because of the morals and mores of the times, and the connections of the two men, these threats would have been carried out. At the very least, Lauren would have lost her little boy to his father. She also would have lost her job, which she desperately needed. Employers didn't care to have unmarried pregnant women around; *married* pregnant women weren't exactly welcomed in the workplace either.

Lauren returned to her gynecologist, begging for the name of an abortionist. He refused, telling her it was wicked to even entertain such a thought. He knew of a couple, he said, unable to have their own child, who would welcome hers. They would pay all the medical bills. All she would have to do was have the baby and hand it over to its adoptive parents at birth.

Lauren tried to explain that she would lose her son if she went through with this pregnancy, not to mention her job. She was caught in a trap. The only way out was abortion, as much as she hated the idea. She pleaded with the gynecologist for just a name or a suggestion, but to no avail. Although abortion was a criminal act from a legal standpoint at that time, Lauren found a practitioner who operated in a clinic with medical instruments rather than on a kitchen table with coat hangers. It was an extremely bad time for her. A loving, tender-hearted person, she was troubled for months after the abortion with nightmares of her destroyed baby crying for her.

One month after the abortion, Lauren suffered abdominal pains which escalated in their severity. She returned to her gynecologist, who was furious when he discovered that she had gone ahead with the abortion. After the examination, he told her that she had peritonitis, a severe infection of the lining of the abdomen, and that he must operate on her immediately. She didn't want surgery and asked if there wasn't some kind of antibiotic treatment that could cure her.

"If you want to live, you'll let me do this surgery," he replied. "I've got to clean you out—uterus, ovaries, everything."

Terrified, she agreed. It was late on a Friday afternoon. The surgery was scheduled for the following Monday and Lauren was told to be at the hospital by three o'clock on Sunday. She went home, cried, prayed, paced, didn't sleep. She desperately wanted more children and hoped to marry again. On the other hand, if she died from this infection, where would any future children be? And what would happen to her little boy?

She said that weekend was the most miserable of her life. On Sunday morning a great calm came over her—she thought at the time she'd gone around the bend—and she simply decided to do nothing. She did not call the doctor, did not call the hospital. She simply did not show up.

Lauren expected to become a great deal sicker. Instead, the abdominal pain lessened until it finally disappeared altogether. Time went by, she met a nice man, they married, and she had two more children.

When she was forty-two, Lauren was diagnosed as having fibroid tumors. She went to three gynecologists, all of whom advised hysterectomy with concurrent removal of her ovaries.

"Although I fought surgery before," Lauren said, "it was different now. I had my children. I *was* tired of the menstrual thing and what the doctors said made sense. Why should I keep something I didn't need anymore? They all assured me I wouldn't miss my uterus and ovaries any more than I would miss an appendix. So I went ahead with the surgery.

"But since the hysterectomy, sex doesn't feel the way it did before. I don't have the longing for physical intimacy that I

72

used to have. It caused a lot of trouble between my husband and myself. We went back to the doctors, who told us, in effect, that I was having mental problems. I spent a period of time in counseling but nothing helped. Things got worse at home. My husband finally left and I didn't blame him. He's a great guy. He deserves a woman who can give him a good sex life. I realize that somehow it was my fault, although I'm not sure how. But at least I have my three children. So I'm luckier than some."

One must wonder at Lauren's statement that her husband is a "great guy." Not all husbands flee when hysterectomy changes the quality of their wives' sexuality. Gerald R. is a corporation attorney in southern California. He and his wife, Betty, had been married thirteen years when Betty was diagnosed as a candidate for hysterectomy because of uterine bleeding. The couple had two children and were contemplating another two when they were told of Betty's condition. Gerald had a consultation with his wife's gynecologist, after which he urged her to go through with the surgery.

"I was afraid her condition could become cancerous," he said.

It took Betty nearly a year to recover from her hysterectomy, which included removal of the ovaries, and even after that Gerald said she felt almost continually exhausted. She no longer seemed interested in sex but when her physician said he had never had a complaint of sexual dysfunction before and recommended a psychologist, Gerald and Betty both went through a course of treatment for six months.

Now Gerald says: "We stopped when it became increasingly obvious that Betty was deemed to be at fault in some way. I know the change in her has something to do with her surgery but I don't know what. As far as I'm concerned, she's my wife, I love her, and our life will always be together. How would I feel if the tables were turned, if she left me because I became impotent?"

Acceptance of her own "guilt" was one of the biggest problems faced by Anne B. As a teen-ager she had overheard health complaints shared by members of her mother's bridge club, most of whom had undergone hysterectomy.

"All I heard was how they didn't have any energy, how awful they felt," she said. "Then there were other remarks exchanged in whispers that I couldn't hear but I was sure it had to do with their sex lives. In my own mind I called them The Hotflash Club and privately vowed that no matter what happened to me, I would *never* be like them."

When Anne was thirty-five she underwent hysterectomy, consenting to the simultaneous removal of both ovaries. She had no plans for marriage or for children; at the time she was totally occupied with her career in chemical research. She said her main reason for consenting was the fact that hysterectomy would be the ultimate birth control. Also, she was pleased at the idea of having no more menstrual periods.

Anne said it took her nine months to recover from the surgery. Then she was horrified to discover that she was tired all the time; she was depressed and had suffered an enormous drop in libido.

When she went to her gynecologist, he prescribed estrogen tablets. Determined not to be like the members of her mother's Hotflash Club, she said nothing about her depression or changes in her sexuality. When she left, the doctor stood up and smiled.

"It's a pleasure to work with an intelligent woman," he told her. "You don't fantasize depression and loss of sexual drive. Smart women are too busy for that."

Anne remained silent, afraid to tell him how she really felt; afraid that he would consider her an unintelligent woman.

Even bright, sophisticated, worldly women have bought into the medical profession's expectation of their sexual and reproductive organs; surely something will go wrong with them, necessitating their speedy removal, and smart women don't suffer any unpleasant aftereffects.

Women find it difficult to talk about the problems connected with hysterectomy. Tatters of prudery hang stubbornly on in the most unlikely places. Probably the height of prudery was reached half a century ago when Lady Gough's *Book of Etiquette* cautioned: "The perfect hostess will see to it that the works of male and female authors be properly separated on her bookshelves. Their proximity, unless they (the authors) happen to be married, should not be tolerated."

Today women explore space and run for the highest offices in the land, but most still feel a certain sense of shame or distaste about their own bodies. Many still are not at ease with their sexual organs. From childhood, they are taught that their "privates" are not quite nice. Afraid that these areas look funny and smell funny, women wash and spray with fragrance, and some shave in an attempt to make these funny-looking parts more acceptable to their partners. One woman said her husband claimed her sexual organs looked "like a piece of old raw liver." The sad part was that she willingly accepted his oafish evaluation.

The realization that many women find it difficult to talk about sexual problems following hysterectomy has prompted some enlightened health care centers to have their personnel make a special effort to pick up conversational clues pertaining to a woman's worries about this surgery. The subject is so sensitive—and the fears so nearly impossible to express to another person—that even highly articulate women hesitate to talk about them.

In a closely related context, that of emotional disturbances suffered by women in their mid- to late forties, it has been found that although 90 percent of all women experience irritability and depression during this time, only about 25 percent bring these troubles to the attention of their physicians.

No wonder gynecologists estimate that no more than 10 percent of the female population suffers severe menopausal symptoms as a result of endocrine dysfunction. But the fact is that gynecologists are *not hearing* from 65 percent of the troubled women, according to studies conducted by psychiatrists Frederick T. Melges and David A. Hamburg.

Why aren't the rest of the women talking to their doctors? Is it because of women's natural reticence about their female functions? Or is it because of what they perceive to be their physicians' insensitivity on those subjects?

The ability to desire and enjoy sexual contact with another human being is one of the greatest gifts of life. Its loss is tragic. Said one woman: "Since I can't enjoy sex anymore, life isn't as much fun. Even the flowers aren't as bright."

One of the most difficult problems concerned with post-hysterectomy sexual dysfunction is the inability or unwillingness of the medical profession to take such female dysfunction seriously.

Molly A., at forty-eight, is a handsome, dynamic woman who has strong ties with the literary and artistic fields. Her second marriage was to a well-known professor some forty years older than herself.

When Molly was forty-five, doctors removed her uterus and ovaries with no thought of possible sexual complications. At the same time, doctors hesitated performing prostate surgery on her husband, then eighty-five years old, fearing the possible loss of his virility!

"I'll tell you what they did to me," Molly told me. "They caponized me."

When a male is involved with a possible loss of sexual interest and powers, physicians give a great deal of serious consideration to the problem. With women, they don't even consider it a problem.

What has caused this unawareness, this blind spot, on the part of the medical profession?

It is the result of what in law is called "the dead hand rule," that those long dead still hold sway, not only over property, but also over ways of thinking, over standards of conduct.

Call it the ultimate sexism or a holdover of old fears. It dates back to the time when a woman was not understood to be a sexual being—or perhaps *feared* as a sexual being—and hence, perceived as a second class citizen at best. She was receiver of a man's name, receptacle of his seed at his express pleasure, producer and nurturer of his young—if she were lucky enough, that is, to be chosen by him for all this largesse.

In one way or another, this sexism still exists and is certainly linked to the education received in modern medical schools.

Over a hundred years ago, students in Philadelphia chased women out of their lecture hall, throwing wads of tinfoil and tobacco quid at them. The year was 1869. Not long after, the men of Harvard resolved to ostracize the first female student, issuing a statement that "no woman of true delicacy" belonged in a medical school. Even Oliver Wendell Holmes, Sr. (the physician, not the jurist), who had outwardly supported an applicant when she approached the faculty for admission, was not consistent with his so-called liberated view of the female. He described woman—not *a* woman, but womankind in general—as a "constipated biped with a backache."

That was over a century ago. How is it today?

Recently, Dr. Mary Howell, the first woman associate dean at Harvard Medical School, sent out questionnaires to women at 107 degree-granting medical schools querying them about contemporary attitudes.

She was "simply astonished at what came back." Now a practicing pediatrician in the Boston area, Dr. Howell found the following:

- Over a hundred years after men had found women unfit to receive medical education at Harvard, present-day professors across the United States were still telling females that "a woman's place is in the home."
- One chief of ob-gyn told students: "A woman doesn't belong in the operating room except as a patient or as a nurse."

- One woman medical student wrote to Dr. Howell: "It is common knowledge that the head of our ob-gyn department disapproves of women medical students. During a lecture on contraception, he flipped various sizes of diaphragms Frisbee-like across the lecture room with vulgar remarks regarding sizes and compared the use of contraceptive foam to a pastepot."

Many doctors' attitudes about their women patients were just as demeaning as the medical school staffs' attitudes toward women students, Dr. Howell found. For example:

- A Chicago gynecologist said: "The only significant difference between a woman and a cow is that a cow has more spigots."
- A gynecological lecturer showed pictures of the vulva, and made obscene remarks concerning its beauty or lack thereof.
- A prominent gynecologist referred to a patient as a "cute trick."
- Another consistently referred to his single middle-aged female patients as "spinsters."
- Another commented: "I'm surprised that women, particularly older women, are sensitive about having a breast removed."
- Yet another described his women patients as "whiny."
- Still another, when queried on the subject of sex drive after hysterectomy, replied: "You can't compare it with a man losing his testicles. After all, a man has to *erect*, he has to *do* something. All a woman has to do is lay there."
- Another referred to hysterectomy as "pelvic house-cleaning" and "taking out the garbage."

These are the attitudes that pervade in much of today's medical practitioners and that scare women away from attempting honest conversations with them. Those women courageous enough to try such conversations are too often given one or more of the following answers:

- Your sex life will not be affected by hysterectomy. If anything, it will be improved.
- Sex may feel different after hysterectomy because of your missing uterus, but most happy, well-adjusted women don't even notice this. (Don't *notice?* How insensitive are women supposed to be?)
- If you're over forty or have stopped menstruating, your ovaries should be removed even if there is nothing wrong with them because they will be damaged by the surgical procedure of removing the uterus. And, don't forget, removal of your ovaries could prevent you from getting ovarian cancer. Why have two operations when just one could clean you out?
- Do not listen to old wives' tales about how hysterectomy can spoil your sex life. Even if the old wives are your best friends, walk away.
- If you have the surgery and later have problems with your sex life, you will need psychiatric help. There's no way that operation could cause such dysfunction. If you claim you enjoyed sex before the surgery, you probably didn't, but just said you did. The operation has given you a good excuse to stay away from sex now. In either case, psychological counseling is needed.

It is a sad but certain fact that while many gynecologists are caring, sensitive people, many more are not. Some male gynecologists suffer from a male contempt of women as valid sexual beings, capable of feeling pleasure in their own right. And there are women gynecologists who subscribe to the same view, having accepted the mistaken concepts about women passed down in medical schools for centuries. For a physician to assert that a woman's reproductive organs have nothing to do with her sex organs shows either abysmal ignorance or an incredible lack of concern for the woman involved.

Dorothy O. and her husband are Mormons. They have three children, two boys and a girl. When Dorothy was thirty-two, she began spotting after her period.

Halfway before her next period was due, she developed a painful backache. The spotting continued. Her doctor told her to keep in close touch; it was possible she had a tubal pregnancy. She doubted this because she had always been extremely nauseated almost from the first moment of pregnancy. One morning she awoke with lancing pains between her shoulder blades and vomited. The doctor told Dorothy's husband to get her to the hospital where he would meet them.

After a few tests, Dorothy was prepped for surgery. The doctor told Dorothy and her husband that she had a tubal pregnancy which had ruptured. She asked if he would have to "take anything out." He replied he'd have to see after he got in there, but it was certain that one ovary and a Fallopian tube would be lost.

She said she remembered begging him not to take anything else out; even if it was necessary, she wanted to be conscious first and have an opportunity to discuss it with him. He promised, patting her hand. As Dorothy was being wheeled into surgery, too foggy with the pre-op shots to say anything, she heard her husband tell the doctor he might as well "clean her all out," that they didn't want more children anyway. Later, when she was conscious and the surgery was over, she was told she had undergone total removal—uterus, tubes, ovaries.

Dorothy's husband assured her it was "for the best," that they wouldn't have to worry about her getting pregnant anymore.

She said that at the present time, five years after her hysterectomy, she suffers from fatigue "constantly." Regarding her sexuality, Dorothy confided that it must be greatly reduced as she hasn't slept with her husband since the surgery, although, she admitted, "I think a lot of that's because I'm still so angry with him and the doctor for getting rid of my organs without even consulting me." She said that as soon as their children are grown, she will leave him.

Lesbian women suffer from the same insensitive response from their gynecologists. Claire W. is a high technology typesetter by trade and a perennial college student, now working toward a master's degree in English. When she heard that I was writing a book on hysterectomy, she approached me and asked if I would be interested in her experience.

"I was married for three years," she began. "It's taken me eight years to recover." The end of her three-year marriage (there were no children) also ended Claire's relationship with men. She met a woman who became first a best friend, then a lover. About a year later Claire had a total hysterectomy. Before her surgery, she and her friend had a close physical relationship.

"I lost all desire for sex after my hysterectomy," she said. "Here I am, thirty-two, and I don't care whether I ever go to bed with anyone or not. In fact, I'd just as soon not."

After Claire's surgery, she suffered from depression so severely she had to quit her job and go into therapy. She said her psychologist didn't understand her problem, but she thinks personally that "it has something to do with my body chemistry being all screwed up after that kind of surgery."

I asked about her relationship with her friend. She started to cry. Her friend needed more than Claire could now give. "She's found someone else. I understand she's happy."

"Why did you have a hysterectomy?" I asked.

"That's a laugh," she said bitterly. "I got three opinions. *Three.* They all told me I had some fibroid tumors and, since I was a lesbian and not likely to have children because of my life style, I'd better be cleaned out. I was afraid of that tumor."

So much of hysterectomy has to do with a physician's attitude, not only about the surgery but about the woman herself. In Molly's case, her doctor's attitude was that her uterus and ovaries could be removed with no thought of possible sexual complications while the removal of her eighty-five-year-old husband's prostate gland gave pause because of possible sexual dysfunction.

In Dorothy's case, her physician evidently agreed with her husband that he had control over her sexual and reproductive organs. She had nothing to say about it.

In Claire's case, all three of the physicians she consulted agreed that since she was a lesbian, she didn't need these organs.

The case of Leslie O. is yet another in which a physician's attitude prevailed. Leslie is a vice-president of a national advertising agency. At thirty-eight she has fought her way up in a highly competitive field, not so much from burning ambition on her part, but because her husband, whom she married when she was nineteen, was never able to earn enough to support two families.

Leslie was thirty-four and mother of four children when a gynecologist told her a hysterectomy was the "only sensible decision" for her to make. She requested a second opinion. The original diagnosis was confirmed. She had a fibroid tumor. Both physicians recommended removal of her ovaries at the time of her hysterectomy. After they explained it all to Leslie, it made sense.

"You're all cleaned up," her doctor said cheerfully the day after her surgery. "In a few weeks you'll be knocking them dead again."

When she saw her doctor for her first checkup, she complained of hot flashes. "Please don't tell me I'm joining the Hot Flash of the Month Club!" she groaned. "I'm not ready for that."

The doctor laughed. "A little estrogen will help."

Leslie was back at work after six weeks. She recalled that about three o'clock every afternoon her energy suddenly deserted her with a sudden gush as if someone had pulled the plug, a not uncommon physical response to major surgery. About nine months later, which was longer than she anticipated, her full strength returned but her sexual desire didn't.

"I guess I went a little crazy," she said. "I can't believe the heartache I could have avoided if only I'd known that loss of sexual desire was to be expected after this kind of surgery. *That* I could have lived with."

At first mystified, then concerned, and finally panic-stricken about her loss of desire and fulfillment, and receiving no supportive information from the several doctors she consulted, she decided, finally, to experiment outside of her marriage. Once the ice was broken with the first affair, subsequent affairs were easy. But it was to no avail. "It always seemed that maybe the next one would work, would be the magical combination. But there was nothing."

One of the agency's minor clients was a professor of English. Leslie found herself drawn to him. When the professor invited her to dinner, she accepted. During this time, Leslie had been visiting a clinical psychologist about her lack of sexual response, with no positive results except a large bill.

After six months of dinners with the professor, he called to suggest dinner at his home. Leslie felt safe and open with him by now. She was in desperate need of a true friend, one who would be undemanding sexually, but to whom she could unburden her heart. During a comfortable pause in their after-dinner conversation, Leslie told him the whole story. She didn't tell him how she had been playing around. He was quiet for so long that she feared she had embarrassed him with her disclosures.

Finally he said softly, "Although I've never married, I've lived long enough to know that there comes a period in a sophisticated woman's life when she requires more sophisticated lovemaking, lovemaking to match her own mental and spiritual growth. The lovemaking of youth, which many men never grow beyond, is all right for youth. It is uncritical, undemanding, except for frequency."

He took her hand. "I have the greatest admiration for you. Let me make love to you. Let me show you what you need."

Leslie said she was so entranced by his offer, so curious about his method of lovemaking, so flattered by his apparent desire for her, that she accepted. In the bedroom, he undressed her slowly, then told her to simply lie on the bed, to do nothing herself, that he would do it all. What followed was slow and deliberate, an approach calculated to drive Leslie to the height of enjoyment. She said: "My orgasm almost tore me apart! Yet, even with the strength of this orgasm, it was like it was surface, a surface thing, rather than deep inside like it used to be. Then it was all over."

Their second encounter was a replay of that first night. Her reaction wasn't so overwhelming because she knew what to expect. Eventually Leslie's affair with the professor died a natural death. After the first novel excitement, she suffered the same sexual dysfunction with him that she did with her husband. She doesn't experiment outside of her home anymore. She said it wasn't worth it. Has she ever come to terms with her loss of sexual desire?

"It doesn't make any difference now," she said. "I have my room. My husband has his. We don't bother one another."

Which somehow is the bleakest answer of all.

Chapter Four

THE
FORBIDDEN
TERM

"Castration," the male gynecologist shuddered. "Please don't say that word. I hate it. I never use it. It sounds so final."

"But isn't removal of a woman's ovaries actually female castration?" I asked.

"Well, yes," he admitted.

"And isn't that what it's called in medical circles?"

Again he nodded. "But we only use it among ourselves. In the medical profession," he hastily assured me. "We never say that to patients. It would be too threatening."

The word castration *is* threatening, the fact even more so. Men wince when they hear it. Most men, when told the title of this book, blink and back away. In some men the reaction is not so marked, but it is there. Women, on the other hand, move forward, hungry to know more.

It is not surprising that men react so dramatically. The concept of castration touches on their deepest fears, represents the greatest insult that can be perpetrated against the male biophysical system. Testicles are terribly important to men. One of the worst things that can be said about a woman is that she is a "ball-breaker," that she can render a man inconsequential as a male person.

In many respects, a man's genitals *are* the man. More than merely a symbol of manhood, they are the very essence, together with his brain, of what he is as a human being.

Why haven't birth control pills for men been successfully developed? The greatest deterrent to research has been the fear that such a pill for men would alter and diminish the male libido. Scientists worry about diminished male sex drive. They don't worry about diminished female sex drive because they don't consider it important.

Why not? They argue that libido is needed to put the sperm where it belongs but that no libido is needed to put the female egg in place. Species continuation, they declare, rests on the libidinous male. One government population official is quoted as putting it this way: "Most women don't have those orgasms you read about anyway. A lot of that Masters and Johnson and Women's Lib stuff is about the extremes, almost the abnormal. I never heard any hesitation based on whether the pill would affect whether a woman could have an orgasm."

In referring to penile implants, devices that artificially restore a man's ability to attain an erection, it is said that the procedure is *more* than an operation. It is the restoration of a shattered ego, making a male a man again.

Male castration is very serious. Recently the South Carolina Supreme Court ruled that male castration is an unconstitutional "form of mutilation" and ordered that three convicted rapists be resentenced because they had originally been given a choice of castration or thirty years in prison. The Supreme Court justices ruled three to two that the circuit court's sentence was void because castration is cruel and unusual punishment prohibited by the state constitution.

In another recent case, a man was awarded $1.75 million when he claimed he became impotent after his Colt six-shooter (the gun that won the west) went off accidentally and wounded him. His wife was awarded an additional $500,000 for "loss of services and companionship," meaning that he could no longer participate in normal sexual relations with her.

Has any husband been awarded a large financial settlement because his wife is no longer interested in sex after her hysterectomy? Has any woman received a financial award for loss of her sexual organs?

Medroxyprogesterone acetate, commonly known by its trade name, Depo-Provera, is a synthetic version of the hormone progesterone. It was originally developed in 1957 by Upjohn as a contraceptive. The United States Food and Drug Administration will not allow manufacturers to market the drug for this purpose because of alleged indications that it may cause cancer, although it has been approved for use in treating cancer.

In women, the drug disrupts the ovulation cycle. In men, it lowers testosterone to prepuberty levels.

In some states it is being used on male sex offenders with long histories of raping women and sexually abusing little girls and boys, to give these men a holiday from their sex drives, allowing them to experience life for a while free of their exaggerated and perverted sexual appetites.

In other states this use is not permitted. Many are violently opposed to this method of treatment, not because of any possible cancer-causing effects, but because they see use of Depo-Provera as "chemical castration," and therefore too heinous a treatment to be visited upon these men. This, despite the fact that the libido-reducing effect of the drug is only temporary, ceasing when the drug is withdrawn.

It would seem that reduction of libido is too serious to be endured even temporarily by male sex offenders, while reduction of libido in castrated women is too inconsequential to be given serious thought—or any thought at all.

The male penis and testicles are of great importance to the male world, and are seen to be so by everyone. Although the female ovaries are just as important to women, they are not seen to be so by anyone except the women who have lost them.

This startling difference in attitudes is illustrated by a personal note. Just before my hysterectomy, when I expressed concern about the effect of the surgery on my marriage, a friend who still possessed all of her organs replied: "Why should you worry about it? Is that all you are to your husband, just a set of ovaries and a uterus?"

Is that all a man is, just a set of testicles and a penis? Why are men's organs sacrosanct and women's expendable?

Is a woman any less than a man, that she can be cut into with impunity, with no thought for the loss of her gift of sexual desire?

This attitude is far worse than the maintenance of a double standard between a castrated man and a castrated woman. It is blatant denial of the existence of a woman's sexuality.

What's wrong with the medical profession? Are doctors too ill-informed, too insensitive, too careless to understand what happens in a woman's body after hysterectomy?

In many ways, doctors are like everybody else. Some *are* ill-informed, insensitive, careless, lazy, too eager for the fast buck—just like any cross-section of lawyers, accountants, dentists, undertakers, computer programmers. For the most part, however, they are dedicated, hardworking people, most of whom really care about their patients.

But in certain significant ways, doctors are terribly different from other professionals.

First of all, they wear halos around their heads that shout Certified Lifesaver. Deep down, where nobody else can see, way below the surface cynicism, most people really think of doctors as gods who walk among men. It's difficult to question a god. How can a woman tell Dr. Jones he was sure wrong about sex after hysterectomy when he's just saved Great-aunt Grace's life?

The pronouncement, "The doctor says . . . ," is almost synomomous in power with that other authoritarian statement: "In the beginning God created the heaven and the earth."

Secondly, most doctors are men. Being men, they are prone to the concept that women's sexual organs are really there for childbearing and male pleasure, rather than simply for women's pleasure. Imperial Roman soldiers carried their swords in scabbards which were called *vaginas*. Romans also labeled the passage out from the female uterus a vagina, thereby decreeing, apparently for all time, that a woman's vagina is significant solely for its abilities to house and please a man's penis and plays no role in providing pleasure for its owner.

Most men also suffer from an innate belief that woman should not be a sexual creature—certainly not the woman who receives the bestowal of his name and the blessing of his seed. While a man may long for passion—fantasizing wild couplings with passionate creatures half woman, half legend—true passion in his mate is suspect. It troubles him. Is he satisfying her? Has she taken a lover? Where has she learned these tricks? Is she becoming a nymphomaniac? Is something wrong with her glands? In their traditional conclaves over poker tables and in hunting parties, men exchange stories of marvelous encounters with female sex fiends. But if one of their number actually has a sexy mate, all the others feel sorry for him. So, if a passionate woman consults her doctor because she has lost her passion after surgery, there could very well be an impasse. Male doctors have male hang-ups.

Thirdly, doctors are products of medical schools which are still rife with sexism and misinformation about women. The intellectual elitism that medicine fosters creates a sense of omnipotence.

The New Our Bodies, Ourselves, by The Boston Women's Health Book Collective, reports:

Women often complain bitterly of the cold, abstract, impersonal or authoritarian doctors. A major study by the Institute of Medicine found that a majority of families were dissatisfied with their doctors and up to half had changed them as a result. These qualities may have less to do with the physician's original personality than with the one-sidedness of her or his training. Similarly vital knowledge needed for optimum patient care—how to evaluate studies and risks accurately, what tests and treatments really cost, how to recognize a patient's rights and identify the ethical issues involved in medical decisions, what patients could do for themselves to prevent illness—is either absent altogether or relegated to the status of an elective. Students get the message: this material is not important.

Discussing the admiration of young physicians for teachers and doctors who command enormous amounts of money as well as authoritarian power, one distinguished medical educator says: "What emerges are physicians without inquiring minds, physicians who bring to the bedside *not* curiosity and a desire to understand but a set of reflexes that allows them to earn a handsome living."

And handsome business it is, indeed. Medicine today in America is a $400 billion a year business, and it is still growing. Physicians are businessmen. They have to be. As in any business that is successful, they must be aware of and expert at promoting their product. They must understand marketing and showmanship and practice it assiduously. Their flashdance steps in the advertising musical must be far more intricate and subtle than those of their retailing brothers who sell sofas and diamond rings and automobiles.

An important part of surgical training is learning to persuade a patient to agree to surgery. The most successful sales technique is a subtle innuendo suggesting what will happen to the patient if she doesn't have the operation. Next in popularity is for the physician to imply that the surgical procedure will benefit the patient even if that possibility is negligible or even remote. Finally, there is the technique of avoidance. The doctor merely avoids informing the patient that there are alternative and less invasive methods of treatment.

Lela J. experienced all three sales techniques. A thirty-two-year-old widowed mother of two, Lela was having irregular periods. Some months she had no period at all; other months she flowed heavily. Her gynecologist did a D and C, found no malignancy but told her she had some uterine polyps and a small fibroid tumor. To Lela, her gynecologist had always been the final authority on anything pertaining to her body. He suggested a hysterectomy and oophorectomy.

"Is it a matter of saving my life?" Lela asked.

"No," her doctor replied. "Not at the moment, anyway. But

one never knows what these things will turn into. And sometimes it happens so fast there's not much time to do anything."

Now Lela was really worried. If anything happened to her, who would rear her children? They were alone in the world, without close relatives.

"It's a simple operation," her doctor went on. "We can remove the uterus and ovaries and you'll never know they're gone. Except that you won't have to bother about menstruation and you will have the finest birth control should you ever decide to enjoy life again." He smiled. "You'll feel like a new woman with more energy than you've ever had before."

Like most women, Lela could certainly use more energy. The idea of no more periods to worry about was appealing, as was permanent birth control. Someday she'd want a relationship again. It would probably happen faster, she told herself, if she didn't have to worry about getting pregnant.

Lela's doctor sold her on the operation. He did not tell her that her condition could have been easily treated without surgery. Now, she regrets the surgery. It is true that she no longer has periods and doesn't have to fear pregnancy. However, her energy is always at a low ebb, she is depressed much of the time. She has met a man whom she loves deeply and will marry; but, she said, she can't enjoy the physical aspect of their relationship as much as she expected to, as much as she could have before her hysterectomy.

Surgery has become so common that most women are too easily convinced that an operation is necessary. Women are an easy sell. Yet medical researchers *themselves* are now suggesting that at least seven common operations—hysterectomy, tonsillectomy, cholecystectomy, appendectomy, cardiac revascularization, gastrectomy, and radical mastectomy—may no longer be necessary or may soon be replaced by other treatments.

Rates of surgery could be reduced by as much as 45 percent with no threats to health if second opinions by physicians were required, according to a 1985 report released by a Senate panel. Nine types of frequently unnecessary surgeries were cited, among them hysterectomy.

The Senate Special Committee on Aging reports that the Medicare system alone could save up to $1.2 billion a year by eliminating unnecessary operations.

In the last decade the number of surgeons has multiplied seven times faster than the general population has grown, while the overall surgery rate has increased four times. It is a fact of life that where there are a lot of surgeons there will be a lot of surgery.

Women in one Maine city are three times as likely to undergo hysterectomies as are women in a neighboring city—not because they have more gynecological problems but because the first city has more surgeons and more hospital beds.

Professors John Wennberg of Dartmouth Medical School and Alan Gittelsohn of Johns Hopkins recently studied 193 separate areas in New England, ranging in population from 10,000 to 200,000. They calculated the rate of surgery, insurance-reimbursement rates, and number of hospital beds per capita. Adjusting for age differences among populations, they then calculated rates of hospital admissions for surgeries in the eleven most populous areas of Maine, Rhode Island, and Vermont. They discovered that the highest hysterectomy rate was four times the lowest hysterectomy rate. Their conclusion: that better health in some communities simply does not account for the contrasts.

The crucial factor, they said, appeared to be the system of medical care in each community; the number of physicians and hospital beds in proportion to the population varied widely.

As to why decisions made by doctors differed so widely community to community, the researchers found that procedures with the most varying rates were the procedures whose risks and benefits to the patients were the least well-established in the medical profession. Their conclusion was that without authoritative standards, doctors are left to disagree in treating the same symptoms. The consumer becomes a guinea pig.

Where there are a lot of surgeons, there will be a lot of surgery. Where there are a lot of internists, there will be a lot of diagnostic tests. The American way of suing has contributed much to this overabundance of medical testing. Some people believe that from a medical standpoint, the best place to live is in a small town with one overworked family physician who's too busy to get experimental.

Gynecological surgery is on the increase in the United States. A growing number of obstetricians are getting out of the baby business to concentrate instead on gynecology. The major reason is the high cost of malpractice insurance, which in turn is based on the enormous sums that juries have awarded to plaintiffs in lawsuits filed against obstetricians.

American doctors pay more than $2 billion a year for insurance against malpractice suits, a cost usually passed along to patients in the form of higher fees. Obstetricians, orthopedists, and neurosurgeons pay the highest insurance fees of all medical specialists.

The risk is highest for obstetricians practicing in New York, Florida, and California, where malpractice suits are most frequent and jury awards are surprisingly generous. If an obstetrician is found guilty of damaging a baby at birth, the jury can award millions on the grounds that the child has been damaged for life. Even if the doctor has been found not to be at fault, he will have to spend $50,000 to $100,000 or more defending himself.

Some fear that without enough patients to go around, gynecologists will be tempted to extract more income from those patients they already have by recommending surgery the patients don't really need. In 1975, in a *New York Times* interview, a Baltimore specialist frankly admitted that it was already happening: "Some of us aren't making a living, so out comes a uterus or two each month to pay the rent."

Chapter Five

DO WOMEN
REALLY NEED
MENSTRUATION?

"I'm going to have a hysterectomy!" stormed Lindsay M. "I'm sick and tired of this mess every month!"

The lovely young woman, just twenty-eight, is a talented artist who lives on a 40-acre farm near the sea in a western state.

"Don't even *think* such a thing," I implored. "You'll regret it the rest of your life."

"Why?" She turned toward me. "We don't plan on having children. Why should I be stuck with cramps and bleeding and crabbiness for the next twenty-five years?"

Why indeed, I thought to myself. But I said, "You could never find a doctor to do such a needless operation. There's nothing wrong with you."

"Dr. Morgan said he'd do a hysterectomy if I really wanted one. He said I'd be a whole lot better off."

No, this was not the 1920s or 1930s or even the 1960s. This conversation took place early in 1985.

A gynecology textbook currently in use in our medical schools states that "if menstruation can be abolished it would be a blessing to not only the woman but to her husband as well." Most doctors feel that after a woman has had the children she wants, a uterus with its concurrent menstrual periods is excess baggage.

Helen W. looked forward to her hysterectomy because it would mean the end of menstruation. "It seemed that every time I went on vacation with my husband or had a really important event in my life, along came my menstrual period at the same time. We already had the one child we wanted, so my having to go through the whole menstruation scene appeared unnecessary to me.

"After my hysterectomy I was surprised to discover that my whole rhythm of life was thrown out of balance. I hadn't realized that my menstrual periods provided 'seasons' for me—certain times of the month when I felt more energetic, other times when I felt more subdued and relaxed and others when I felt sexy. Without my menstrual period each month, every day is the same. I knew about some alternative therapies before I had my hysterectomy but I opted for the surgery mainly to get rid of my periods. I would never advise another woman to go ahead with hysterectomy for that reason."

What is menstruation? Does it have value in a woman's life as a physiological function in and of itself? Does a woman need the organs from which it springs after her children have been born?

Yes, a woman needs menstruation. It is a lodestar in her life, providing a sense of psychic direction, of monthly renewal, giving her personal nomenclature. She needs the organs that produce menstruation just as surely as a man needs his penis and testicles long after their ultimately fleeting function of fertilization have been performed. They are part of the individuality of each woman, just as a man's genitalia are part of his own individuality and personal feeling.

The uterus and ovaries are hormone-producing as well as structural organs, which is why a large number of women suffer so many problems after their surgical removal.

As living creatures, our first experience of life is the smell and taste of our mother's menstrual blood. At our birth, her blood is on our lips and at our nostrils, its fragrance inhaled with our first breath. The scent, the flavor and, in some cases, the sight of menstrual blood is the first and most potent imprint we receive.

Yet this headwater of birth and of female being, rich with the most ancient of symbolisms, is considered by many to be unclean, a mess, a drag, a pain in the neck and elsewhere. It is referred to as the "curse," the "wrong time of the month," and as "being on the rag," among a host of other even less appealing epithets.

The ancients believed that a menstruating woman was to be avoided at all costs. Pliny warned: "On the approach of a woman in this state must [new wine] will become sour, seeds which are touched by her become sterile, grass withers away, garden plants are parched up, and the fruit will fall from the tree beneath which she sits."

He reported that menstruating women in Cappadocia were walked about the fields to preserve the vegetation from worms and caterpillars.

Native Australian women having their menses were forbidden to touch anything that men used. This menstrual superstition was so strong that cases have been recorded in which a husband, discovering his wife lying on his blanket during her period, killed her and then died of terror himself within a two-week period.

Aristotle said that the very look of a menstruating woman would take the polish from a mirror and that the next person looking in it would be bewitched.

In some eastern countries, on the other hand, menstruation was regarded as sacred. The first menstrual discharge was considered so valuable that prepubescent marriages were held in order that the first ovum might not be wasted but rather fertilized because it was thought to be the purest and the best.

But usually the menstrual period was regarded by men as a cyclic occurrence which was abhorrent and disgusting. It was a time when women leaked evil excretions. In some cultures, the menstrual discharge was regarded as polluting, exceptionally debilitating, even physically dangerous to men. During menstruation women were forbidden to prepare food and were rigidly confined to special quarters that men never entered because they believed these quarters were always polluted.

A girl's puberty ceremony was the greatest ritual occasion in the entire culture of the Indians of the American Northwest and the Apaches of the Oasis. The ceremony, held during the flow of menstrual fluid or just after it had ceased, lasted for several days and included much feasting, singing, and dancing. Everyone in the local community was invited by the parents of the girl and even outsiders were urged to attend.

In northwestern California, elaborate annual rites called World Renewal Ceremonies are still performed. For countless years Indians have held these rites to renew the contaminated world. When asked what polluted the world and made these ceremonies necessary, investigators were told that menstrual fluid was the principal offender. Female physiology is tremendously important to these Indians. While the girl's puberty rites themselves are of modest proportions and the subsequent menstruations of women are little discussed, the tidal flow of women is the center about which the greatest ceremonies of these societies revolve.

There is a substratum of beliefs and practices, common to many cultures, that the menstruant is in a state of close contact with the supernatural which may harm her or others if she does not behave properly. She must be secluded; must avoid contact with hunters, fishermen, gamblers, shamans, and priests—all of whom are especially susceptible to harm at this time. She must diet in order to avoid illness or bodily disfigurement; she must abstain from meat so as not to spoil the hunting success of the men who killed the game. She must not touch her body with her hands, lest she catch a skin disease or lose her hair, but must use a stick provided for that purpose; and at the end of the taboo period she must be bathed and dressed in new clothing.

All cultures dominated by men, both historically and at the present time, have strict taboos against sex at the period of the month when female blood flows. Sex at such a time will make monsters, they say. Sex at any other time (times when pregnancy can occur) is all right. This is a universal taboo and one from which we can infer that the only worthwhile part of a woman's nature is that concerned with conception and childbirth.

The creation of children is only one part of human joy, and one that many women choose to forgo altogether. Equally important to female fulfillment is sexual love.

For centuries, women knew what it felt like to conceive, carry, and bring forth a child. After the medical profession made an illness out of childbirth, drugging women into a state of oblivion during the process, women forgot. Soon it became the fashion to exchange horror stories (particularly in front of a first-time expectant mother) about lengthy labors, horrible pains, the excruciating sacrifices endured to bring a child to life.

I grew up on stories like these. When my oldest daughter, Mindy, chose natural childbirth, I was horror-stricken. I spent a miserable eight months worrying, and trying to talk her out of such madness.

But the day came, in my home, and I was able to watch the miracle, emotionally overcome by the outpouring of mystery and beauty and love—and by my daughter's deep communion with her body. She felt pain, but she knew it was productive pain. She understood its purpose.

Being an adopted child myself (and not knowing I was adopted until I was twenty-nine), I never knew my beginnings. There was a lonely blank. I had apparently started from a dead end. But when I held my granddaughter, still wet from my daughter's womb, I felt for the first time the rising tides of genesis. I knew who I was. I knew some part of me would go on in this tiny Heather, my darling, who, being *grand*, was somehow more than daughter. The pain of unanswered questions, of unknown beginnings, was soothed. I didn't know where I had come from. But I knew where I was going.

This was the most consciousness-raising experience of my life. By being so in tune with her body, my daughter enabled me to learn how to become in tune with myself. I will always feel a deep gratitude to Mindy for this gift of love.

There is another time for total and rewarding communion with one's body, a time that represents yet another ancient wisdom lost in our high-tech society—a woman's experience of her own selfhood during menstruation. Surely there was great wisdom passed from one generation of women to another in those huts to which menstruating women were banished long ago. Ethnographers say men never set foot there. It was more probable that they were not permitted to do so. The menstruation huts were sacred to women and their knowledge, to the exchange of menstrual and fertility mysteries, to the mystery of womanhood itself.

There is evidence that groups of women in the past were able to exert influence over the events of conception and birth by techniques of deep introspection. It is known they were able to menstruate at the same time of the month. This phenomenon is known today in communities of women who have close intellectual ties.

Menstruation is one of the functions that makes woman miraculous. It is a resurrectional function: without it the human race would not exist. And it is tied inextricably with the act of sexual intercourse.

In David's *Song of Solomon,* one of the most stirring statements ever written about physical love, his Love says:

I am the rose of Sharon
And the lily of the valleys . . .
As the apple tree among the trees of the wood,
So is my beloved among the sons . . .
Also our bed is green . . .

Her Prince responds:

The joints of thy thighs are like jewels,
The work of the hands of a cunning workman.
Thy navel is like a round goblet, which wanteth not liquor;
Thy belly is like an heap of wheat set about the lilies.

Sources are prudish about the true translation of the word navel. Clarke's sourcebook says it is "too sensuous." As if anything can be too sensuous in the physical love relationship. Margoliouth translates it as "the bowl of the moon." Sometimes *navel* means body. Moffat translates it as waist instead of navel, with the apparent meaning of pelvic basin.

Lap is closer to the true meaning, say Penelope Shuttle and Peter Redgrove, in their lyrical book, *The Wise Wound.* They assert that what the word actually means is, as in Shakespeare, pudendum, vulva or cunt. The 1952 Revised Standard Version of the Bible reads:

Your navel is a rounded bowl that never lacks mixed wine . . .

To the man, the mixed wines of the *Song of Songs* would mean his semen mixed with the woman's juices in her lap or pudendum. This wine of the vagina is the sexual fluids that flow and mix. The Biblical poem proclaims the vigorous sexuality of two people in deep physical love with one another.

A woman herself has two kinds of mixed wines. Ancient sources called these the River of Life and the River of Death; the clear or white flow at the times when a child could be conceived and the red flow of menstruation, when it is most unlikely that conception can occur.

Aristotle saw the universe as a partnership between mind and matter, with matter being shaped by an insubstantial power which could imagine and bring into material existence an infinite selection of forms or ideas. His belief was similar to that expressed in the Hebrew Old Testament where a spirit brooding on all possible forms moved over the shapeless matter and drew it out into the familiar things of nature.

In his great work, *On the Generation of Animals,* compiled in the fourth century B.C., Aristotle made it clear that this cosmological process was repeated on a small scale in the conception and growth of living organisms. He thought that the male sperm was the spiritual agency which conjured limbs and organs from the menstrual blood provided by the female, just as mountains, rivers, and continents had been molded from formless matter by the soul of the universe.

If a woman is not impregnated, she menstruates. Some call this the weeping of a frustrated womb. Many physiologists and doctors, and some feminists, feel that a uterus is for growing babies, and without that function, it is a useless, redundant organ. They regard menstruation itself as a sickness.

Conception and nourishment of the unborn, however, is only one part of the spellbinding role played by a woman's sexual organs.

A woman's whole body participates vigorously in her menstrual rhythms. Every month, all through the month, she goes through a series of fantastic bodily changes of orchestrated sensitivity. Some of the events that are continuously occurring include changes in:

- Sex hormone levels in blood and urine
- Buccal, rectal, and vaginal temperatures
- Basal metabolism
- Blood sugar
- Endometrial glycogen
- Water retention
- Body weight
- Pulmonary vital capacity
- Alveolar CO^2 concentration
- Arterial oxygen pressure
- Blood acidity
- Serum bicarbonate
- Heart rate
- Erythrocyte sedimentation rate
- Differential blood leucocyte counts
- Platelet counts
- Serum protein
- Vitamins A, C, and E concentrations
- Bile pigments

- Blood adrenalin
- Urine volume
- Thyroid and adrenal function
- Electrical skin resistance
- Pupillary size
- Psychic activities
- Pain threshold
- Vaginal cytology
- Skin color and permeability
- Breast size and sensitivity
- Composition of the cervical mucus secretion and citric acid content
- Viscosity and gravity of the urine
- Work performance
- Electroencephalogram readings
- Olfactory, visual, and auditory acuity
- Ability to walk a tightrope

It is not possible that organs so deeply involved with the fiber of a woman's body and with the chemistry and electricity of her brain would not be missed in subtle as well as obvious ways, would not cause deep and radical changes if removed. To give credence only to the ovulation aspect of the menstrual cycle, as physicians do when they suggest a uterus is not needed after a woman's children are born, is to limit the role of woman to just this one function.

Is the curse, then, really a curse? Is there anything good about it? Most women, in their wish to ignore the phenomenon altogether, remain totally unconscious of the changes brought about by this monthly occurrence. They do not realize the mind-body links which are so invisibly potent. They ignore the physiological events of the cycle that links the body's roots to the mind in a physical manifestation of the old allegory of the Tree of Life which has its roots in heaven and its branches and fruits within the ground. Those women who suffer from premenstrual syndrome (PMS) are aware of changes, but only in a negative way.

Menstruation is a time whose value modern women have neither recognized nor appreciated, a time when healthy women may draw on capacities not related to the values of ovulation and childbearing—values that belong to the other side of woman, the side devoted to independent thought and action.

It can be a time for spiritual withdrawal from the outside world, of personal renewal, a time of quiet, of taking stock, an Indian Summer of reflection and shared love, a monthly season of solstice before the duties of dawn and summer break once more.

Different energies are available to women at this time, energies calling her to look within—to perceive, accept, and nurture the child that is herself rather than a separate child she would expel from her body.

Actually the menstrual cycle is made up of two cycles—the ovarian and the uterine—the two interlocked by a complex system of nerve and hormone pathways.

Nothing is isolated. All changes interact with all other changes. There is no independence, only interdependence.

The three phases of the ovarian cycle are the follicular, when the capsule containing the egg is ripening; ovulation itself, when the egg is expelled and swept into the Fallopian tube; and the luteal phase, when the remnant of the egg capsule becomes a ductless gland and secretes progesterone. All this activity is preparation for pregnancy.

If pregnancy does not occur, the uterine cycle—which is the phase that is known most popularly as the "menstrual cycle"—is entered. There are three phases to the uterine cycle: the proliferative phase, wherein the uterus builds a new lining for itself in response to estrogen secretion by the ovary; the secretory phase, when the uterine wall grows enormously thick in response to the secretion of the corpus luteum in the ovary; and the discharge phase, in which, if no fertilization takes place and the ovarian secretions suddenly decline, the uterus lining is expelled.

It is a harmonious symphony. The ascension of one level

stimulates the production of another substance which in turn regulates the first level and initiates yet another process.

One of the greatest myths is that menstruation is an abnormal condition, something that goes wrong every month. In fact, it is something that goes *right* every month. Extremely painful menstruation is the exception rather than the rule.

For decades women were told that the unpleasant physical and emotional symptoms some suffer before menstruation were "all in your head." It was humiliating to be disabled by a phenomenon everyone said was psychosomatic. Now medicine admits that a woman's premenstrual pain is caused by a biochemical abnormality. They have put a nice label on the condition—premenstrual syndrome, or PMS—which now makes it all right to suffer from. As many as nine out of ten women suffer a variety of unpleasant physical and emotional symptoms *before* menstruation. One or two women in ten suffer from severe PMS.

While psychological factors may increase a woman's discomfort, they do not cause it. The true cause is a biochemical imbalance. The most common signs and symptoms of PMS in any of its forms include swollen and tender breasts, bloating of the abdomen, fatigue or depression, anxiety, constipation, skin eruptions, headaches, and cravings for sweet or salty foods. For many women, such symptoms begin a week before the period starts and disappear a day or so before menstruation begins.

No single treatment is effective for all women. Doctors may prescribe various drugs for the severe cases. Progesterone may be administered, as well as medications termed antiprostaglandin agents, which relieve symptoms caused by the body's overproduction of prostaglandins—potent chemicals that trigger cramps, headaches, nausea, and other problems. Progesterone is so powerful that, as a partial cause of PMS, it can cause the body to retain over six pounds of water, a whopping two-thirds of a gallon.

There is evidence that more women who conform to traditional roles suffer from PMS than do women who diverge from these roles. The divergers who do suffer during their cycles tend to do so from cramping pains in the uterus itself. There are indications that PMS sufferers benefit from accelerated dreaming, particularly about family and childhood experiences. Uterus cramp sufferers benefit from increased sexual experience on both the mental and physical levels.

Women who are not afraid to have sex during their menstrual periods report peak sensual experiences, with far more orgasms than at other times. The texture of intercourse is entirely different in subtle as well as in obvious ways. Orgasm at this time causes an ejaculation of blood from the cervix into the vagina.

The uterus itself, abundantly supplied with consciously sensory nerves and filaments is, at menstruation, an exquisitely responsive sense organ. Always open to stimulation through the genital organs, at menstruation the uterus rewards its owner with exceptionally deep and throbbing ecstasy.

The female body feels more open and ready for sex than at any other time. Men feel a rare specialness at this time, a sense of the woman presenting to them a unique offering of herself. Part of this is a continuation of the kindness extended to a woman by her partner when love is made just before the onslaught of her period, when she is heavy and crampy, thereby easing the flow to come, when the act may not be as much for the partner's pleasure as it is to soothe and comfort her body.

Numerous studies have shown that most women feel the height of sexual desire during their menstrual periods. Custom has conditioned them to hide this fact. If a woman masturbates at no other time during the month, she is likely to do so during menstruation.

Heterosexual love made at this time should be gentle and persuasive for, without practice, the raw and open uterus may react with pain. Sexual stimulation should be gradual, building slowly to an unforgettable feast of the senses.

Many lesbian women seem to be more at ease with lovemaking during the menstrual period, recognizing that it is a time for joyous sex. Heightened responsiveness plus the physical aspect of extra wetness and warmth is acknowledged and appreciated.

When a woman is capable of menstruating, she is in tune with the tides of the universe. The great currents and tides of the oceans move in rhythm with the seasons. Sensitive women feel these tides in their bodies. Perhaps they feel the enormous pull of the moontide—that vibration that is greatest at new moon and solar eclipse, a time when the sun's force and the moon's force are in line and their gravitational powers are combined. If a woman opens the doors of her consciousness, she may experience these tides. When the menstrual tide is stopped by surgical interference, the tides cease. A great unnatural calm overtakes the female body.

Women need their menstrual cycles. They are refreshed and renewed by them. Once a month, menstruation makes the world new again. And women certainly need their organs of reproduction, even after menstruation has stopped.

Chapter Six

HORMONES AND HYSTERECTOMY

"You don't need your uterus," the gynecologist told Penelope W. "And as far as sex goes, that's all in your head anyway."

After the operation, Penelope thought she was going crazy. "Things that never bothered me before started irritating me beyond belief. I wanted to cry all the time, and I never used to cry. The whole world seemed as if it had turned against me, so I started to fight back, beginning with my husband. I got so hard to get along with that I lost my job of eighteen years. I couldn't stand my husband, in bed or anyplace else. Until I had the surgery, I had always needed him sexually.

"The worst was one night when I was coming home from a class in painting and a policeman stopped me to tell me I had a tail light out on my car. I thought he was stopping me to give me a ticket. I didn't give him a chance to say anything. I just tore into him, screaming and yelling and even trying to hit him. Then I collapsed and sobbed. He was very nice. He escorted me home and suggested to my husband that I should see a doctor. Which I did the next day.

"The doctor said it was hormone trouble and put me on estrogen. It took several weeks to get the dosage balanced out, but after he did, I felt like a human being again, although it didn't have any effect on my sexual desire. If my husband and I have sex once every six months now, that's a lot. It used to be four or five times a week. I guess there's some hormones they can't replace."

When doctors say sex is all in a woman's head, they are right to a certain degree because the brain is the conductor of the sexual symphony, controlling the functional activity of the ovaries by acting through the anterior pituitary gland. Pituitary hormones stimulate target tissues. When the target is a gland, as in the case of the ovaries, one response of the target organ is the secretion of its own hormones. Thus, hormones from the pituitary stimulate both the follicular growth in the ovary as well as the secretion of estrogens from the ovary.

The lack of feminine hormone feedback in the pituitary gland causes many severe problems in castrated women. Hormonal difficulties can range from slight to severe. Some can be balanced with the use of artificial hormones, others cannot. Such imbalance can cause loss of libido, unusual behavior, depression, chronic fatigue, and abnormal aging.

Woman's hormonal past is bizarre. During the hunting and gathering period, which occupied 99 percent of mankind's evolutionary history, mature females were either pregnant or nursing for most of their lives. Few lived to the age of menopause. The reproductive period lasted less than two decades.

Today, women have a reproductive life of more than thirty years, during which only one or two pregnancies may occur. Even these will probably not be followed by a prolonged period of nursing with the consequent suppression of ovarian cycles. As a result, the brain and the rest of the modern feminine body are subjected to repeated surges of hormonal stimulation and withdrawal, far more numerous and more closely spaced than the tissues and organs were evolved to withstand.

If thirty-three years were to intervene between menarche and menopause, and if there were no interruptions due to pregnancy or lactation, a contemporary woman could expect to experience no fewer than four hundred menstrual cycles in her lifetime. If she had three children and nursed each one for six months, she would still experience over three hundred menstrual cycles.

By contrast, a woman of prehistoric times possibly had no more than fifteen years of reproductive life and nursed her surviving young for at least two years, which would then allow time for no more than ten periods of menstruation in her lifetime.

The biological fact is that civilization has given women, along with their right to compete with men in everything, a physiologically abnormal status with regard to periodic fluctuations in the secretion of their ovarian hormones.

What are these ovarian hormones? What do they have to do with a woman's brain? With her sexuality? With her perception of herself as female?

According to the classical definition, a hormone is an exotic and wonderful chemical agent synthesized in one tissue, secreted into the vascular system, and then carried to a distant site of action in the body. The so-called sex hormones are androgens, estrogens, and progestins which are secreted by the testes, ovaries, adrenal cortex, and, in pregnant females, the placenta.

Attention was first directed to these compounds when it was discovered in the mid-1800s that castrated young roosters stopped mating and their accessory sex tissues began to disappear. But when given testicular grafts, their combs would grow and they would resume mating.

It was not until the present century that researchers fully realized that the gonads (the ovaries in females, the testicles in males) exert such effects because of their chemical secretions. And it was not until the 1930s that estrogen, progesterone, and testosterone were chemically identified.

The isolation, identification, and sythesis of the gonadal hormones led to numerous studies in the United States during the 1940s on the effects of gonad removal and hormone replacement. One of the most important discoveries was that the administration of any particular hormone does not insure stimulation by that hormone; it may be metabolized in the body and take on an entirely different form, which in turn exerts its own specific effects.

Late in the 1930s, evidence began accumulating that the brain plays a major role in the regulation of sexual function, doing

---

so in two major ways: controlling the functional activity of the gonads or ovaries by acting through the anterior pituitary gland (adenohypophysis, or AP); and mediating sexual excitability, or libido, and modulating sexual reflexes by responding to gonadal hormones and to sensory stimuli.

Hormones originate in a tiny section of gray cells wedged in the middle underside of the brain, the hypothalamus, which is Greek for "under the inner room." In that area, somewhat smaller than the average prune, a supply of a triggering chemical called LHRH gets jammed into a series of narrow, downward-stretching channels, falling half an inch until the pituitary gland is reached. Representing the lowest boundary of the brain, this small gland, slightly larger than a pea, dangles from beneath the brain at about the level of the sinuses.

This pituitary gland has been called the leader of the endocrine orchestra—endocrine meaning all those glands that help orchestrate what we are by secreting their responses to life into the bloodstream. Small but mighty, the pituitary is a complex structure that secretes ten different hormones. Part of the pituitary's structure includes what is called the anterior pituitary (adenohypophysis) which produces the two gonadotropic hormones—FSH, a substance which stimulates ripening of the ovarian follicle and LH, which induces ovulation. In addition to these two gonadotropins, the anterior pituitary secretes other hormones including prolactin, which facilitates milk production by the mammary gland; ACTH, which acts on the adrenal cortex; TSH, a thyroid stimulating hormone; and GH, known as the growth hormone.

The intermediate lobe of the pituitary, called the *pars intermedia,* secretes two melanocyte-stimulating hormones. The neurohypophysis, or *pars nervosa,* produces oxytocin, which influences the contraction of the uterus and plays a role in milk letdown; and vasopressin, which has antidiuretic as well as vasopressor (producing a rise in blood pressure) effects.

The first indication that pituitary hormones might influence the brain came from repeated discoveries of these hormones in hypothalamic, or brain, tissue. Later, a variety of studies indicated that these hormones could influence the electrical activity of the brain, the release of FSH and LH, and the synthesis and release of gonadotropic-releasing hormones.

The brain, the pituitary, and the ovaries are continuously linked in their functions. Pituitary and ovarian hormone secretion patterns are closely linked in time with changes in sexual behavior, in the vaginal smear pattern and in uterine weight. Here's how it works.

The primary pathway involves the stimulation of the pituitary by the brain and the subsequent stimulation of the ovaries by ovarian hormones which are secreted by the anterior pituitary gland in response to brain stimulation. The pituitary exerts feedback effects upon the brain while hormones secreted by the ovaries exert feedback influences upon both the pituitary and the brain.

In sexual arousal, the triggering chemical is squeezed down into the pituitary from the hypothalamus overhead. Once this occurs, the pituitary pushes another chemical along the narrow blood vessels that run around its edge. The hormone is sucked in, and once within, begins the ride that takes it all through the bloodstream. This two-step action, according to David Bodanis, author of *The Body Book,* starts automatically once every hour and goes on in these chambers and tubes behind our noses hour after hour for all of our adult lives.

The second chemical rides along with the bloodstream as it rushes down the neck, trickles across the lungs and flows past the elbows. It does not stop until it encounters the only cells in the human body that will utilize it—the cells in the female ovaries and the male testicles.

In women, when this triggering chemical pours into the ovaries, or ovary, or piece of an ovary, it locks into certain cells, forcing them to let loose with all of the ovarian hormone, or estrogen, they have on hand and then to get busy manufacturing more. A woman then feels the beginnings of sexual arousal as her body begins to ready for possible sexual intercourse. As long as even a portion of an ovary remains, this feminine hormone feedback goes on.

113

In 1955, twenty-four-year-old Charlotte T., mother of a two-year-old son, suffered a sudden excruciating pain in her lower back one Sunday afternoon while her husband was working in the yard of their home. The pain was so intense she couldn't walk, so she crawled to a window and called for her husband to come inside.

Seeing the condition she was in, he immediately phoned their family physician who instructed him to bring Charlotte to the hospital. Tests were taken, and Charlotte and her husband were told she was suffering from a ruptured appendix, a ruptured ovarian cyst, or a ruptured tubal pregnancy.

It proved to be an ovarian cyst. When Charlotte's abdomen was opened, the pressure had been so great that blood and pus shot to the ceiling of the operating room. After the surgery, the doctor showed Charlotte's husband the cyst, a grayish sac about six inches long and ruptured on one end. Charlotte's left ovary was removed at the same time.

Ten years later, Charlotte developed a tubal pregnancy that ruptured. Part of her right Fallopian tube and half of her right ovary were removed.

She said she had no diminuation of libido or any problems with depression and fatigue until the rest of her remaining ovary was removed at the time of a hysterectomy two years ago.

"As long as I had even a piece of one ovary, everything worked fine," she said. "Now, I have problems. The most obvious one is that sex isn't a pleasure anymore."

Ovarian hormones cause a female to be attracted to males and to exhibit various behaviors which engage the male's attention and arouse him sexually. They are what make an embryo into a boy or a girl. If the fetus is to be a girl, female sex hormones will be swirling around by the seventh week in the womb, causing the smooth skin at the base of the abdomen to develop into the labia lips and the clitoris. In a male fetus, testosterone will cause the same tissue to shape itself into the scrotum and penis. Even a mild lowering of sex hormones will stop the libido in both sexes. The hormone androgen would be most likely to stimulate sexual desire and satisfaction, but in order to have such a stimulating effect on a woman, androgen would have to be administered in such quantities that women would experience unpleasant masculinizing effects such as deepening of the voice and the growth of facial and chest hair.

About five percent of a woman's sex hormones is made up of the male hormone testosterone; men have about the same percentage of the female hormone estrogen. The pattern of hormone secretion in the female is cyclic, which is why some women get more benefit from monthly hormone shots than from daily pills. In the male such hormone secretion is tonic, or regular, reflecting the differentiation in the brain which takes place early in development and which is under hormonal control.

Both sexes produce both estrogen and androgen, although in different proportions. Hormonal sex differences are a matter of ratios, not absolutes.

Experiments on the rhesus monkey by B. J. Everitt and J. Herbert revealed that without ovaries the rhesus female lost sexual interest in the male. At the same time, her nonodiferous vagina failed to attract his interest.

In both rhesus monkeys and in man, the occurrence of sexual behavior is less closely tied to endocrine events than it is in the lower mammals. Females of both species engage in sexual intercourse throughout the menstrual cycle. There is strong evidence, however, that sexual behavior and hormone secretion are closely tied. According to extensive studies done by N. M. Morris and J. R. Udry, intercourse and orgasm are far more likely to occur at the time when estradiol secretion is at its maximum. These findings were based upon daily reporting by human subjects.

Although many glands influence behavior directly or indirectly, the androgens, estrogens, and progesterones are the major performers in the sexual symphony.

Men who have had their testicles removed have empathy for women who have gone through hysterectomy.

Steven P. is one of those men. Five years ago, a specialist informed him that he had cancer of both testicles and they would have to be removed.

Steve's way of dealing with the shocking news was to tell no one. His wife of twenty-odd years had recently left him, and had moved to another city. Two of their children were grown and living elsewhere. The third went with his mother.

Now, at forty-five, Steve had to rethink his life. For many years he had owned an industrial electrical business. In the late '70s Steve and his wife vacationed in Wyoming and fell in love with the area. Then they discovered a motel-lodge for sale. So smitten was Steve with the prospect that he overlooked some important details. But he forged ahead, turning the management of his lucrative business over to an old friend and employee.

It was a huge mistake. After a run of incredibly bad luck, Steve lost the motel to its former owner. His financial problems were staggering. Steve's wife returned with him to their former home where she stayed just long enough to pack her things before their home was seized, then grabbed a plane for San Diego. "I'm sorry," she said, "but this business with the house was the last straw. I don't wish you any more bad luck. But, please, just stay out of my life."

And then the doctors told him the bad news. The surgery was done. Steve says it was extremely difficult to accustom himself to not having the weight of his testicles, the *awareness* of them, suspended from his body.

Then he began having what he calls "real weird problems. The hair on my chest disappeared and my voice got high. I'd actually cry at the drop of a hat. I got so depressed I thought it would be best if I killed myself. There were days and days when I didn't even get out of bed except to go to the bathroom. Now and then I'd take a job, just enough to keep eating.

"Finally I decided there was no way I could go on like this. I called the oncologist, who sent me to an endocrinologist. After some tests, they started giving me a series of shots. Pretty soon I was feeling like a new man. My chest hair grew back, my voice deepened and I stopped weeping and feeling so depressed. I know this is what a lot of women go through—not that they lose chest hair—but the awful depressed feeling. I tell you, it's hell."

Now Steve feels pretty good—except when it's time for a shot. Then he gets grouchy, depressed, exhausted. He goes for his shots every two weeks, more frequently if he feels he needs them.

Hormones are known to affect the senses of smell, taste, touch, and hearing. For example, an adult woman who possesses her ovaries can readily detect the odor of exaltolide, a substance with a chemical constitution similar to that of civet. She cannot smell it when she is a child, and she cannot smell it after the menopause or the surgical removal of her ovaries. A man can never smell it unless he is given an injection of estrogen.

The most important way in which hormones produce concurrent effects upon behavior is to induce temporary changes in brain function. Increase or decrease in estrogen or progesterone affects emotional responses in most women. Estrogen replacement therapy helps untold thousands of women achieve a sense of well-being. Unfortunately, it does not help with libido.

Alice M., thirty-five, is a professional photographer who had undergone hysterectomy including removal of both ovaries when she was thirty-two. She claimed she wouldn't be able to function in either her professional or private life without hormone replacement therapy. Following is an excerpt from her diary:

> April 10—It is one of my porcelain days. I move carefully, or not at all, to keep from breaking. My head aches, my bones hurt, my skin burns, my ears feel plugged, my mind is fuzzy. I don't hear well. I lie down and sink into deep sleeps. I know if I do something about

it today, it won't get too bad. If only I could force my-self to get dressed! I must. In one more day the killer depression will be on me. I need a shot.

Got my shot at four p.m. Within an hour I was myself again.

Many aspects of human behavior are more deeply influenced by hormones than present investigational methods are capable of revealing.

Important new research now being done may answer some of women's problems. The Institute for Advanced Biomedical Research, the nation's first institute for studying the molecular biology of the brain, is being built at the Oregon Health Sciences University in Portland, Oregon.

Headed by Edward Herbert, Ph.D., whose team has made some of the most important brain discoveries in the past dozen years, the group will include geneticists, molecular biologists, endocrinologists, protein chemists, cellular neurobiologists, and immunologists.

One of the team's studies now in progress at the University of Oregon, Eugene, is the role of the brain peptides, a recently discovered group of brain hormones that are involved in a bewildering array of effects, from stress reactions to runners' high, depression to obesity, schizophrenia to drug addiction. Presently under intensive study is the question of how peptides help our bodies control pain, and the role they play in sleep, temperature regulation, cell growth, sexual cycles, learning and memory.

For women who have undergone removal of their ovaries, the proper balance between estrogen and progesterone therapy is a *must*. Some women take hormone replacement in the form of tablets.

Others find that tablets don't work for them; that the most effective replacement therapy is in the form of shots administered once every three to four weeks.

One world-famous endocrinologist has stated that if this replacement therapy is not handled properly by a woman's attending physician, that woman would have grounds for a malpractice suit.

Studies are needed regarding hormonal effects on men and women, including speed and magnitude of penile erection or vaginal lubrication, duration and intensity of physical stimulation sufficient to produce orgasm, number and strength of muscular contractions involved in sexual climax, duration of postorgasmic refractory period and so on.

It would also be of value to measure frequency of intercourse and/or masturbation under fairly constant conditions. Some of these variables have been examined but rarely in combination with differences in hormone levels.

The mechanisms through which estrogen influences sexual attractivity vary from species to species, but odor and taste of the female's secretions and excretions are involved.

Estrogen changes the chemical composition of perspiration, urine, and vaginal secretions. Males are sexually stimulated by smelling and tasting these products of the female body. For some primate species, estrogen changes the appearance of the genital region and the swollen "sex skin" serves as a visual stimulus to males.

The estrogen-induced sexual attractivity of female primates is depressed by progesterone. One study of a small group of married women revealed that husbands were less likely to initiate sexual relations during the period immediately after the wife had ovulated, and was beginning to secrete increasing amounts of progesterone.

Hormone deprivation is a horrible feeling, truly unimaginable by those who have not experienced it. Dorothy C., a forty-three-year-old midwesterner who raises prize cattle, has taken hormone shots once a month since her total hysterectomy ten years ago.

"When the scare about estrogen causing cancer was publicized, I didn't stop my shots," she said. "I didn't care *what* estrogen was supposed to cause. The quality of my life would be so loathsome without supplemental hormones that I'd rather be dead anyway."

Contemplation of suicide is common with hormone deprivation or imbalance, in both sexes. All things seem tragic, all people hateful. Inappropriately administered hormones can be tantamount to a death sentence.

The late Alan Turing, an acclaimed British mathematician, code analyst, and computer pioneer, developed a machine that broke "Enigma," Germany's most secret code, thereby providing the Allies with advance information on German battle plans that helped win World War II. Turing was also a homosexual, a fact he did not attempt to hide. In 1952 he was arrested and found guilty of "gross indecency," a term commonly used in those days.

Rather than serve time in jail, Turing chose the offered alternative—medical treatment which consisted of large doses of the female hormone estrogen. The treatment rendered him impotent and caused him to grow womanlike breasts. The inappropriate doses also caused him to develop severe untreatable depression. On June 7, 1954, this national hero committed suicide by eating an apple dipped in cyanide.

Considering how the female body is made, how the organs function, it is not surprising that women who have surgically lost their ovaries do not feel the overwhelming sexual desire they once felt. What is surprising is that the medical profession apparently has not understood the simple concept that with the removal of a woman's ovaries, the chain of desire is broken. Something most important and very necessary is missing. The synchronized flow between brain, pituitary, and ovaries has been destroyed. It isn't that a roadblock has been set up—the road itself is gone.

Chapter Seven

SEX AND HYSTERECTOMY

"The earth moved," said Maria, the heroine of Ernest Hemingway's immortal *For Whom the Bell Tolls,* in describing her orgasm.

The earth *should* move during lovemaking. That's what natural, satisfying, good sex is all about. Good sex need not be complicated. It is simply the ultimate expression of closeness between two people. It is the physical and spiritual merging with another for whom we feel great affection, ardor of soul, closeness of mind, and fullness of heart. It is the joining with our other self, making what is incomplete complete. Good sex flows naturally, springing from a watershed of *feeling* between two people. Some say that sex is not all there is to a relationship. Perhaps not. But it can certainly make or break one.

At the physiological level, sexual desire starts the same way every time. We see or think about a special person, think of a haunting memory, smell a fragrance, read erotically moving words. Reactions to any of these stimuli pass along the nerve-cell circuitry throughout the body, rushing into a group of nerve cells contained in a ring formation near the bottom of the brain. This is the limbic brain system, formerly called the rhinencephalon, the "smell brain," which is now known to be profoundly involved in human emotions.

In animals, the stimulation of this region leads to faster breathing, increased rate of heartbeat, meaningful gestures with shoulders and hands, facial grimacing, erections, grooming activities, stomach rumbles and, in some cases, impulsive, yet hesitant aggression. In inhibited humans, it merely shoots out brain signals that will eventually produce broader sexual feelings. We attempt to subdue stomach rumbles.

Sexual arousal is first shown outwardly by changes in the eye. As sexual interest rises, blood pressure builds and the eyes' pupils open wider. In less than one-fifth of a second they grow from a two millimeter pinpoint to eight or nine millimeters. Tiny spoke-shaped muscles located in the colored part of the eye and reaching into the pupils cause this change. Simultaneously, six muscles in the eye socket pull the eyeball from one position to another and the normal rate of blinking which is once every six seconds or so becomes slower. To prevent the now more exposed eyeballs from drying out, an automatic mechanism pumps down on small tear-containing sacs located beneath the skin just behind the eyes. These sacs send out a minuscule spray of tears, giving lovers in moments of passion that well-documented dewy-eyed look.

In tests, a number of men were shown two photographs of a woman, each photo identical except for the fact that the second picture had been touched up to enlarge the pupils. Almost all the men preferred the second picture, without knowing why. When a man said he preferred the second picture—the one of the woman with enlarged pupils—the man's pupils enlarged also. This response to a response represents an ultra-refined body language.

Inside a woman's body, long-term arousal is provided by the sex hormones that are always circulating around in small amounts. Behind every quick arousal, every speculative glance, a marvelously convoluted chain of hormone-associated events is taking place. A hormone originating in the brain begins the ride in a woman's bloodstream, not stopping for anything until it encounters the only cells that will make it halt and grab hold— the ovaries. Sweeping into the ovaries, this triggering chemical forces the ovaries to pour out all of the ovarian hormone, or estrogen, on hand and then to begin making more. The ovarian hormone, in turn, surges through a woman's body, raising general sexual interest and assisting the body to ready tubes, tissues, and organs that will be called into play later if a sexual encounter occurs.

If such an encounter *does* occur, a woman's body—under the right kind of stimulus—will go through a series of splendid accelerations, an impressive physiological chain of events that proceed, one after the other, as inexorably as the movement of the tides.

For a woman, all the physical delights of orgasm happen on the bottom of a sheet of muscle that indirectly wends its way up the center of the abdomen to the level of the lungs. The labial lips are attached underneath to a sinuous ligament that stretches inward to form a ring around the bottom of the uterus—the cervix—then on to the very back of the pelvic bones. The smooth muscle of the uterus is controlled by the same sympathetic hypogastric nerve as the muscle of the male reproductive tract which, when it contracts, moves semen into the urethra before orgasm. Some researchers feel that the lit-' tle-studied contractions of the uterus during orgasm may be the counterpart of seminal emission in the male. The swelling, tightening, and pumping that occurs at the bottom of the uterus vibrates all the way up a woman's body, making orgasm a unique whole-body experience.

There are two types of female orgasm, although some women haven't learned to experience both. These are the outer, or clitoral orgasm, and an inner, visceral orgasm. The contractions of the clitoral orgasm are controlled by the pudendal nerve which originates from the second, third, and fourth sacral nerves. The visceral, or thoracolumbar, orgasm is mainly character- ized by contractions of the uterine and the periurethral glands controlled by the pelvic alpha-adrenergic nerves. Many women experience a "mixed" orgasm, with the visceral orgasm adding depth and texture to the clitoral orgasm. Other women expe- rience them separately.

The erogenous sensory zone of the inner orgasm is not lo- cated in the clitoris but in the anterior wall of the vagina, next to the periurethral glands, and presents the same fibroelastic texture as the male's prostate gland. Some women report emitting a sort of orgasm fluid that is probably produced by the periurethral glands. This fluid contains a high level of prostatic acid phosphatase and resembles the prostatic component of semen; both the periurethral glands in women and the prostate in men share a common embryologic origin. The female emission takes place after an inner, visceral orgasm, which follows stroking of the erogenous anterior wall of the vagina. Individual variations of this glandular system could explain the inconsistencies of the emission in women.

Some women say hysterectomy makes no change in their sexual desire and fulfillment. The fact is that much of sex after hysterectomy has to do with sex *before* hysterectomy. If, for example, a woman had a condition that made every sexual encounter painful, and her hysterectomy removed the cause of the pain, sex will be better for her. It doesn't hurt anymore.

Sexual awareness, appetite, and depth of feeling vary with women and with their partners. One woman said: "After eighteen years of marriage I thought I knew all about sex. I loved my husband. There could never be another man for me. Then my husband died. After several years I met someone else and to my surprise fell deeply in love with him. Sexually, I have never before felt such pleasure. I would never have known it was possible."

There are women who have a feeble appetite for sexual pleasure. Patricia M. is a lab technician with a midwestern medical clinic. Ten years ago she had a total hysterectomy including removal of both ovaries. She is quite vociferous on the point that such a surgery could not possibly have an adverse effect on a woman's sex life—it hadn't on hers. Later, she said that it had been ten years since she'd had intercourse, although she is married. Obviously, for her the operation *had* made no difference in the sex life she neither had nor desired.

Thousands of women who do suffer sexual loss have been sent to psychiatrists, many of whom, not realizing the true nature of the problem, counsel them inappropriately. One leading psychiatrist said: "I've treated thousands of women, many of whom had severe problems with sexual dysfunction. In my ignorance, it never occurred to me to ask them about their operations. How many other psychiatrists are out there like I was? Now I see a whole different dimension."

One has only to look at the literature on sex and hysterectomy to realize the lack of understanding. Fred Belliveau and Lin Richter write, in *Understanding Human Sexual Inadequacy,* "A woman who has had a hysterectomy will sometimes have painful intercourse afterward. Masters and Johnson cite three major causes of pain after this operation: the stitches may have been placed so that the penis hits the resulting scar; a woman whose ovaries as well as uterus were removed may not have been given replacement hormones which would keep the pelvic tissues soft; and a woman who has not been properly reassured may feel that she is less of a woman since she can no longer have children. It is especially important for any woman who must have a hysterectomy to be reassured that her sexual drive and ability to have orgasms will not be affected. She should, in fact, feel better after the corrective operation, lose any unconscious fears of unwanted pregnancy, and have more sexual interest than before."

After hysterectomy, with the shock of reduced or vanished libido, many women feel there is no way to regain this formerly ecstatic experience. But there is. When good sex has been a joyous, *needed* experience between a couple, and the woman is robbed of her desire for it, of her ability to feel or desire to give pleasure, she needs to be able to turn to someone for practical advice and understanding. Across the country groups of castrated women are meeting together, some with sexual therapists, in an effort to overcome their problems. There *is* hope: marriages or relationships *can* be salvaged.

Naturally, sexual appetites differ. One woman and her husband don't have intercourse often, but when they do, it lasts most of the night. The only interruption is when he gets up about three in the morning to smoke a cigar. To some, this might sound exhausting. To her, it's wonderful.

Another woman's husband ejaculates the moment he touches her. This could be a problem, but this couple has worked out a system whereby, following his ejaculation, he uses a vibrator on her until she is satisfied. She says he has become very skillful.

Another man has become adept at oral sex, pleasuring his partner in this way until her orgasm, when he enters so that her clitoris and vagina will have something to pulsate against. Without that, she says, the hard pulsations of orgasm would be painful for her.

A postoperative hysterectomy patient suffering from some form of sexual dysfunction must answer the important questions: What was sex like for you before your surgery? What is it like now?

The following outline can be helpful in answering those questions.

1. Present age.
2. Age when hysterectomy was performed.
3. Type of hysterectomy: uterus only removed; uterus and ovaries removed.
4. Heterosexual or homosexual.
5. Questions you had about hysterectomy before surgery.
6. Questions you now have following surgery.
7. What your doctor told you about hysterectomy before surgery.
8. Speed of vaginal lubrication before hysterectomy.
9. Speed of vaginal lubrication after hysterectomy.
10. Duration and intensity of physical stimulation sufficient to produce orgasm before hysterectomy.
11. Duration and intensity of physical stimulation sufficient to produce orgasm after hysterectomy.
12. Any change in partner's technique required to produce orgasm since hysterectomy.
13. Number and strength of muscular contractions involved in sexual climax before hysterectomy.

14. Number and strength of muscular contractions involved in sexual climax after hysterectomy.
15. Duration of postorgasmic refractory period before hysterectomy.
16. Duration of postorgasmic refractory period after hysterectomy.
17. Frequency of intercourse before hysterectomy.
18. Frequency of intercourse after hysterectomy.
19. Frequency of masturbation before hysterectomy.
20. Frequency of masturbation after hysterectomy.

If your desire has diminished or you no longer derive as much pleasure from the sexual act as you did before your surgery, remember these points:

You are not crazy.

Your marriage or relationship is not on the rocks (though it may become that way if you don't take time to understand what is happening to your body).

You are not getting too old to enjoy sex. Nobody gets too old. One man said that many years ago as a young person in France he had sexual relations with three women—a young girl of nineteen, her forty-year-old mother, and her sixty-eight-year-old grandmother. Which one did he enjoy the most? He said the grandmother was the most satisfying partner, not only pleasuring him the most, but deriving more pleasure herself from the act than either of the two younger women.

You are not alone with your problem. There are thousands of women in the same situation.

Another important question is: Do you still want good sex? If the whole idea now seems rather ridiculous, or too much bother, forget it. You probably won't be successful. Your attitude will play a great role in your success or failure. But if you long for the spiritual as well as the physical fulfillment that good sex with a desired partner can bring, there are ways to re-create a rewarding sex life.

"Use it or lose it!" is a warning that old-timers believed to be true regarding a variety of activities, but especially with regard to sex. Researchers have proven that it is easy for people to kill their own sexual proclivities by simply stopping sex.

Don't try to hide what's happened to you. Don't pretend. Talk to your partner. Tell him how you now feel. Put aside any inhibitions you may have and explain to him how your desire for sex has changed since your surgery, how your needs have changed. Don't let him wait and wonder what has happened to you.

Talk. The things that cause the most trouble are the things that seem too ridiculous or too embarrassing to talk about. Tell him that you still want him a lot but he'll have to make the overtures. He'll have to get you in the mood.

Try to eliminate distractions. Try a special weekend trip to a country hide-away or fine hotel that has blissful memories for both of you. It goes without saying that you *do not* bring along kids, other family members, or another couple. Or maybe just chase everyone out of your home for a weekend, lock the doors, pull the draperies, disconnect the telephone. Think back to the days when it was all new and exciting. Did you want other people around? To what ends did you go to get a little privacy?

You may have to work at this, especially if your relationship has already deteriorated to the point where your partner is totally convinced that you never again want anything of a sexual nature. You may have to rise above remarks like: "Don't tease me, honey. I know you're not interested anymore, so let's just forget it, okay?" Or, even more devastating, "Sex? What's that? It's been so long I've turned myself off. I'm not sure I can get interested again."

He may think your lack of interest has killed his sex life. Imagine his delight to discover that it can be born again! But don't wait too long.

After you've gotten his interest, remind him of the days when all it took was a glance and the two of you couldn't find a bed fast enough, when your desire was so great you didn't even want to waste time with foreplay. You may startle him for awhile, particularly if you were not given to talking about sexual matters in the past. Men can be modest creatures. You must explain to him that you want the feelings of old, but that you are unable to achieve them without his full understanding of what your body needs now. If you don't tell him, he won't know.

Some women experience vaginal dryness after hysterectomy. Where formerly a woman may have complained of too much lubrication, she may now be so dry that hand caressing or any attempt to penetrate by the penis will be unpleasant or even painful. In many women, penetration will be impossible. After this kind of surgery, anything that hurts is simply going to hurt. It isn't going to "hurt good" as in new sex for the young.

Explain to your partner that this doesn't mean you don't want him. It's just one of the physical abilities you've lost. Be frank with him about the dryness. Maybe part of your drawing away has been because you can't lubricate as before. Ask his help. Tell him you want to love as before and he is the one you want. To correct the dryness problem, some women use saliva. Others report that a water-soluble lubricating jelly, which can be purchased at any drugstore without a prescription, best simulates the body's natural juices.

Talk to your partner about touching. A lot of men are not too good at this. When men masturbate, for example, sex therapists say they go right for the genitals but when women masturbate, they like to touch their bodies a great deal first. If men are not informed, it's only natural for them to think that the direct assault is all right. Particularly after a hysterectomy, women need even more generalized touching than before.

Touch is the first step in a fulfilling sexual union. You may think your skin is little more than a husk to be painted, plucked, tanned, and decorated—simply an outer package that holds the rest of you together. Actually, it is one of your most important organs, with functions that are far more complex and varied than even scientists who study the skin imagined only a few years ago.

In addition to being a bulwark, a container, a temperature-controlling system, a rich energy depot, a vitamin and lubricant producer, a vehicle for sensing the outside world and a self-renewing coverall, the skin communicates with the brain through incredibly sensitive nerve endings. Spread out, your skin, which is the largest organ you have, would be about the size of a single blanket. It contains ten million or so nerve receptors. It needs stimulation!

So talk and touch. Open your heart. Someone did a survey about touching and found that in Europe, when friends meet on a street, they touch each other a hundred times an hour. Americans touch each other only three times an hour!

Perhaps you will need to start by touching yourself in private. Some women advise getting totally alone, setting up an atmosphere that is the sexiest for you. Perhaps music, maybe reading something first that really used to turn you on. Fantasize. It won't hurt you and it certainly won't hurt anybody else.

Play gently with your breasts, manipulate your nipples slowly and, if you begin to feel a small desire, apply lubrication liberally to your genitals. Then gently massage the labia and the side, not the head, of your clitoris. This may be done with your hand or with a vibrator. When you feel the urge for penetration, insert the vibrator and explore the upper reaches of your vaginal canal, using whatever motion or speed feels the most desirable. Hysterectomy has shortened your vaginal canal and it no longer has the vertical give that it had when you were in possession of your uterus.

Many women revealed that they have discovered a certain area in the upper reaches of the vaginal canal, usually on their right-hand side, that has a great deal more sexual sensitivity then any other part except for the clitoris itself, and that desire builds if that spot is stroked with soft pounding motions. This is the inner, or visceral, source of orgasm—separate from the clitoris. Some said it was like a second clitoris. You will know by exploration which "side," so to speak, of the vaginal canal responds to this sexual thrust. Maintain this action, withdrawing every now and then to massage the side of the clitoral head. Many women say that the climax is somewhat different than before but unbearably intense, nevertheless. Some women prefer to have their partners do this initial exploration for them. Others opt for absolute privacy, later directing their partner's hands and penis into the right thrusts and strokes.

Kate E., thirty-five and the mother of three children, underwent a hysterectomy which included removal of both ovaries when she was thirty-three. She said her husband, Tom, was very loving and supportive during all of her problems with sexual dysfunction following her surgery. Before her surgery, Kate remembered reading a novel about a woman who could no longer reach a climax. The fate of this unfortunate fictional character stayed in Kate's mind and when she and her husband were making love she would sometimes deliberately try to prevent herself from reaching orgasm, just to see what the experience would be like. She was unable to do so, and always wondered how a woman making love could not automatically have an orgasm.

When Kate could no longer enjoy sex in the old way after her operation, it was Tom who suggested that she experiment with her body. "Kids do it all the time," he told her. "That's how they find out about themselves." Kate experimented alone because she was too shy to have her husband join her at first.

"It was about a year after my operation that I started," Kate said. "For a long time, nothing felt very good. But my husband encouraged me to keep at it. Gradually, things started to feel good again. I found a spot at the top of my vaginal canal that felt like another clitoris. I hadn't even known it was there. When my husband joined me, he was very slow and tender. The first night I had an orgasm without artificial assistance we celebrated with champagne. I still don't have preliminary desire. He has to do a lot more work than he did before, but he says it's worth it to see me enjoying sex again. It's different. But it's good."

One young woman reported that before she married her husband she found vaginal orgasm impossible—though she had had extensive pre-marital sex with him. He could bring her to orgasm only by manipulating her clitoris with his hand, the head of his penis, or his tongue. She said she didn't know whether she believed in vaginal orgasm or not, until an outspoken and much-admired aunt told her she didn't know what orgasm was until she had experienced the deep vaginal kind, preferably in concert with a simultaneous clitoral orgasm.

Being inventive and naturally curious, she experimented, not with other men, but with herself, to discover her own body's capabilities. She used a candle to bring herself to clitoral orgasm, and just as the spasms were beginning, she would thrust the candle deep against her cervix. With each experimentation, she gave more attention to the cervix and less to her clitoris until she was able to come to complete orgasm with just the candle moving against her cervix and no overt attention to her clitoris whatsoever.

"That taught me how it could be," she said. "Next time Bob and I were together, I didn't even let him touch my clitoris. I had him penetrate immediately. We both wanted each other so much we were ready anyway. I could visualize the mouth of my cervix against the head of his penis. I felt a terrific spasm and it was like the cervix was actually opening up to grab his penis. That's the way sex was for us all the time after that until I had my hysterectomy. Then I had to learn all over again."

Different methods work for different people. Some women said that during their "retraining period" with their partners they use the Masters and Johnson technique of lots of touching with no actual penetration. In fact, they imagine a stricture *against* penetration, such as fantasizing that they are virgins and are not "permitted to go all the way." By denying penetration, they find they are building up physical desire.

These exercises will take time and practice. But remember how you loved the practice when you were just starting out?

Lucille C. is a psychologist. At forty-one, six months after a second marriage, she underwent a hysterectomy which left her with what she calls a "sexual anesthesia." Lucille wasn't altogether surprised with her medical legacy as she'd had a number of women patients complain of loss of libido. She and her husband were very much in love and they had open lines of communication with one another. She determined that her problem was physical, not mental or emotional. The couple talked it out.

"Look," Lucille told him. "I won't be initiating sex any-more because I no longer feel any desire. But that doesn't mean I don't love you. I love you intensely. I'm going to have to re-learn sex. Let's do it together."

How are they getting along in the bedroom?

Beautifully.

Sex after hysterectomy *will* be different. With love and work and care, it can be very rewarding. The earth *can* move again for the castrated woman.

Chapter Eight

MEN AND HYSTERECTOMY

Besides a woman's physician, there are two parties to a hysterectomy—the patient and her sexual partner.

Hysterectomy is certainly a male partner's business. Second to women themselves, old-fashioned men suffer the most. These are the men who are devoted to their women, whose sense of love and loyalty prevents them from seeking sexual satisfaction elsewhere. They, too, are in sexual jeopardy. Many of these men eventually lose their own sexual powers in a sort of sympathetic response. Virile men can become impotent, and frequently do, when they have mates who have been robbed of their libido.

A man naturally expects his partner to be incapacitated for a time following the surgery, but after her convalescence, he expects her to feel much better than she did before.

Sometimes this happens. But in too many cases it's just the opposite. Instead of a partner who is lively, energetic and eager for sex, he now has a mate who is exhausted, depressed, suffers from debilitating bone and joint problems, is far less interested in sex, has less intense orgasms (if she has any at all) and, if she forgets her daily estrogen pill or monthly shot, is prone to restlessness, insomnia, scalding hot flashes, and tears.

If the man is led to believe before the woman's surgery that hysterectomy is a convenience, a necessary pruning, a sort of reward to a woman for having produced her children—if he is not aware of the possible physiological effects of such surgery—both man and woman can be in serious trouble.

Lack of knowledge about posthysterectomy syndrome on the part of a man can be as debilitating as the syndrome itself, but in a different, insidious way. For example, if a husband has been told by his wife's physician that there is no medical reason for her sudden lack of interest in sex, it is only natural for him, not knowing any better, to suspect that his wife no longer finds him sexually attractive.

He is even more mystified than she by the changes in their relationship. He may decide that the best way to avoid the problem is to stop attempting sexual relations. Eventually he may begin to shun his wife in bed. What sensitive man wants to continually push himself on an unresponsive woman?

Or, tired of being questioned about the changes in her reactions, *she* may stop accepting him. With each failure, the couple is convinced they have a problem—a greater problem each time—but they don't know what it is. Gradually, they may stop touching and, after a while, stop talking.

A man can be just as emotionally devastated as a woman who fears her partner is no longer sexually interested in her. Sexual desire is a fragile, mysterious thing. It can burn white-hot for reasons known only to the couple themselves and can be stilled by lack of interest. Just as men come in varied shapes, sizes and colors, so do they range emotionally from those who give their posthysterectomy women the utmost love and encouragement to those who say, "If I can't get you pregnant, sex is no good for me."

Unfortunately, Nathan A. fits into the latter category. "I know it probably doesn't sound too good, but after my wife, Emma, had five children she needed a hysterectomy. They took her uterus but not her ovaries. She was the same afterward but I wasn't. I just couldn't have relations with her. I think it was because I knew I couldn't get her pregnant anymore. I'm remarried now. We take precautions because we don't want any kids but deep down I *know* I can get my present wife pregnant if I want to."

Fortunately, most husbands are like John C., who was both sorry and relieved when his wife, Edith, went into the hospital—sorry that she had to undergo the discomforts of surgery but relieved that she was having her uterus and ovaries out.

John was forty-two; his wife, thirty-eight. They had been married for twenty years and had two daughters in high school. John had encouraged Edith to have the hysterectomy. He knew how she disliked the bother of her monthly periods. He had talked with his wife's physician and, although he didn't mention it to Edith, he deeply feared that his wife's small fibroids might become cancerous. John's aunt had died many years before of ovarian cancer and it was too easy for him to visualize Edith going through the same nightmare. When the doctor suggested he might as well take the ovaries, too, to avoid further surgery, John encouraged Edith to have the entire procedure done.

After the surgery, Edith had problems with fatigue and depression; both disappeared when she began taking estrogen, but flared up again immediately if she forgot to take her pills. Although she felt much better after the estrogen therapy, her sexual desire was greatly diminished. John took time off from his business in order to take Edith on vacations, hoping that getting away from her everyday life would solve her problems and put the joy back into their marriage. So far, nothing has helped.

Could this problem end their marriage?

"Of course not," John said. "She's my wife and I love her. I'm not saying I won't some day have sex with another woman. After all, there's nothing wrong with me. But it would have to be very discreet. I would do anything to help Edith and I wouldn't do anything to hurt her."

A husband can be either totally removed from his wife's dilemma, believing that such medical matters are between her and her doctor only, or he can play an important role in her decision for or against hysterectomy. In many cases, his advice and feelings can provide the deciding factor.

Many physicians talk with the husband alone without the wife being present while the decision for or against hysterectomy is being contemplated. Others talk to husband and wife together, creating a sort of togetherness or camaraderie— warriors against the woman's misery.

Edward R. said he was drawn into the warrior's mystique. "My wife and I had a conference with her physician about the hysterectomy he felt she should have," Edward said. "My wife's problem was heavy menstrual periods that left her exhausted at the time, but nothing she didn't recover from in a day or two. When I questioned him he said there was no indication of cancer in any of my wife's tests. But he did say that something like cancer can spring up almost overnight and if she had her organs removed, we wouldn't have that worry hanging over our heads.

"He said, 'You know, Ed, no matter how liberated women are these days, we men still have to take care of them, watch over them. If she were my wife, I wouldn't hesitate a minute in scheduling her for surgery.'

"My wife had already been sold on the operation so she didn't have much to say. She was looking forward to getting rid of her periods. But I asked if there was a treatment instead of surgery. The doctor said he supposed there were different kinds of treatments but they were all time-consuming and since my wife was already forty-five, why not get rid of everything and not worry about it anymore. Then he looked at me and said, 'You don't fool around with an abcessed tooth, do you?'

"By the time we got out of there, I felt like the doctor was St. George and my wife's insides the dragon. When I took her to the hospital, I felt like the knight in armor seeing his lady through a bad time. She had both her uterus and ovaries removed. Afterward, she seemed like a different woman. She doesn't care much for sex anymore but the doctor told me that was normal for a woman of her age."

138

The type of doctor who is treating a man's wife will have an enormous effect on the final decision for or against surgery. If the doctor is one who believes that a woman's organs are disposable, that every woman needs a hysterectomy after she's had children, he will be a major factor in converting her husband; men are as much in awe of the medical profession as are women. If the doctor subtly hints, or declares outright, that his wife's condition *could* become malignant, there probably isn't a man in the world who would voice an objection to the surgery.

So what should a husband do? He should expect his wife's physician to be entirely open about the subject of hysterectomy, telling it the way it is. He should expect to hear that, especially when both ovaries are removed, his wife may experience the usual posthysterectomy syndrome including possible depression, fatigue, and sexual dysfunction. He should read as widely on the subject as he can and encourage his wife to do the same.

Bruce K. and his wife, Mary, are both computer programmers for the federal government. "When she was told she needed a hysterectomy," Bruce said, "she and I researched all the popular literature we could find. According to that, it was a surgery with no particular aftereffects, no more than having one's appendix out. But a friend who works in the medical school library in the city where we live helped me research the actual medical facts. After that, Mary and I together made the decision that she would not have the surgery. The operation had been prescribed for a uterine fibroid tumor. That was two years ago and Mary's tumor hasn't grown at all. Not only does Mary feel great, she's expecting our first child in two months."

If it is imperative that a woman undergo hysterectomy, her partner can be a source of comfort and strength. Under no conditions should he make any reference to her being any less of a woman or sexual being before she goes into surgery. Afterward, if she is not getting the help she needs in the way of supplemental hormones, he should see that she goes to another doctor. If she is left with sexual dysfunction of any kind, he should not nag her about it but, rather, set up counseling for the two of them with an expert sex therapist.

He will have to be warm, loving, understanding, and supportive. He, himself, may need help from a mental health clinic or a psychologist. The sooner both of them can verbalize their mutual problem, the sooner they will be on their way to resolving it. Sexual enrichment is an area of life that belongs to both men and women. A woman makes a tremendous mistake when she thinks: If he really loved me, he'd know without my telling him. Why? A man is not a mind reader.

And a man makes a similar mistake. He doesn't realize that the woman's conditioning has been that under no circumstances does a woman tell a man that something's wrong sexually because such knowledge would cause him to be impotent or to become angry and find another woman. So the woman pretends that nothing is wrong and the man pretends that he doesn't notice that something is wrong. A man can play an invaluable service by encouraging dialogue.

In recent years, men have been permitted to become knowledgeable about and participate in their wive's experience of pregnancy and childbirth. They are taught how to be supportive during the nine months of waiting, and helpful during the delivery, in direct as well as subjective ways.

Perhaps now is the time for an expanding of awareness, for husbands to be equally participatory in the matter of their wives' hysterectomies—not in the surgery itself, but in all matters pertaining to the experience. After all, hysterectomy has to do with that part of a woman's body that has produced their children and has participated actively in the growth of the couple's physical expression of love.

Chapter Nine

HISTORY AND HYSTERECTOMY

Most contemporary women do not question why their sexual and reproductive organs are considered so disposable by the majority of the medical profession. It all started a long, long time ago and it had a lot to do with power.

Woman and her ability to reproduce were the objects of reverence and worship, beautifully typified by a four and a half inch figure about 27,000 years old. An exquisite little fat lady, her head is covered with tightly curled hair. There are tiny bracelets on her wrists. Her hands and feet are comparatively small but her breasts and buttocks are abundantly there. She was carved in limestone by the loving hands of a Cro-Magnon or Upper Paleolithic artist in the days when the Carpathian Mountains were glaciated, when a mammoth could graze at the foot of a glacier a mile high.

Today she is known as the Venus of Willendorf, named after the village, four miles from Vienna, where she was discovered in 1908. A glyptic carving, she is one of hundreds found from France to Siberia. One, discovered in Czechoslovakia, was formed from clay and ground bone made long before such materials were used to make pottery. One found in Siberia was fashioned of ivory. Yet of all the ancient glyptic carvings, the Venus is the only one that is anatomically correct; the others are highly stylized. The carvings represent some of the earliest examples of art, proving that those who made them had a much richer culture than we have wanted to give them credit for. It is noteworthy that all-male religions have produced no religious imagery and in most cases have positively forbidden it. The great religious art of the world is deeply involved with the female principle.

These ancient peoples worshipped Woman the Healer, Woman the Mother, and Woman herself. We know from skeletons discovered from that era that they were probably not aggressive, hence not fighters. A hunting and gathering society, they knew things contemporary man has forgotten—the strong need, for example, to be cooperative rather than warlike. To ancient man, woman was miraculous. She gave him the pleasure of her loins; she created life within her own body and brought it forth from herself. With her potions and unguents, she healed. It was natural and fitting that those who gave life also sustained life. This feeling of awe, of reverence, of love for womankind shines forth from the little Willendorf Venus.

Woman as healer and object of worship is older than history. In ancient cultures, medicine was the prerogative of woman. She took care of her clan or her local community in birth and in death and for most of the time in between. But the role of women as healers is one that has been ignored by medical histories. We are led to believe that doctors and healers must be men, and that this is the way it always was.

The true history of medicine began with women. The earliest recorded explanations of disease were religious, and medicine and religion were so closely intertwined that it was impossible to separate them. The deities who created life or commanded death were also responsible for health and sickness.

One of the first of all creation stories—and there are many—is this:

There was a garden of pleasure in Sumer, which had four rivers, including the Euphrates and Tigris. The great mother goddess Ninchursag allowed eight beautiful plants to grow in this garden, although she forbade the inhabitants to eat them.

Enki, the water god, defied Ninchursag and ate from them

142

and she, angry about it, condemned him to death though she did not expel him from the garden.

Enki fell ill, eight of his organs were affected, and his strength began to fail him. But a fox was able to persuade Ninchursag to save Enki from death. She then inquired about his suffering and created one healing deity for each of his sick organs.

Being female, she was merciful. The Sumerians believed that Ninchursag, the goddess of life, was responsible for health and childbirth. The Assyrian goddess Ishtar was both mother and goddess of health. Isis, the great goddess of the Egyptians, was also their physician.

In those societies, a woman who was priestess/healer was required not only to know the properties and attributes of the healing deities and the appropriate prayers and incantations but also to have an extensive knowledge of botany, minerals, and animal derivatives used in medical prescriptions. The Sumerians, Egyptians, and Assyrians had an impressive list of drugs for treating specific diseases; they ranged from pills and suppositories to lotions and ointments.

The priestess/healer was paramount in the societies of Sumer, Assyria, Egypt, and Greece until about the third millennium. Many of the Egyptian queens were notable physicians: Queen Mentuhetep (2300 BC), Hatshepsut (1500 BC), and Cleopatra (100 BC). Drawings on the walls of ancient Egyptian temples and tombs often illustrate women in their role as priestess/physician, and the writings of Diodorus, Euripides, Pliny, and Herodotus testify to their eminence.

In Sumer, there were many kinds of priestesses whose importance in the economic, political, cultural, and social life of the country was enormous. Both healing and business were conducted in the temples. Archeological evidence indicates that the earliest examples of writing were discovered at the temple of the Queen of Heaven in Erech in Sumer over five thousand years ago. Writing was developed there by women.

The first gynecologists were women who were subcontracted, as it were, as midwives by the priestess/physicians, who were limited in number, high in rank, and too busy attending the sick who presented themselves at the temples. These midwives were responsible women who could be trusted to proceed according to the correct cultural and religious practices. The midwives of both Sumer and Egypt were specially educated and trained. The Ebers Papyrus indicates that their knowledge was quite advanced and included not only techniques for handling childbirth and abortion, but a whole range of problems from breast cancer to prolapse of the womb.

These midwives represent the first example of specialization within the medical field. It implied no inferiority on the part of the midwife nor rivalry with the priestess, yet it was a division with resounding implications for the future.

The violent introduction of the Indo-Europeans into the cultures of the East was marked by the emergence of a powerful male god worshipped by the invaders. In Assyria and Egypt, stories of creation were rewritten, and male deities began to acquire an equal, if not superior, position to female deities.

The primacy given to women in the original creation stories began to disappear. By the time of the 18th dynasty in Egypt (1570–1300 BC), women had been relegated to the role of temple musicians and no longer enjoyed even the status of clergy.

The introduction of men into medicine changed the nature and meaning of medical practice for all time. Medicine began to develop independently from religion, becoming anti-mystical. Gone were the gentle incantations and soothing balms of the priestess/physician, replaced by the surgeon's blade. Just as the development of anesthesiology in the mid-1800s made the business of surgery widespread, so the practice of embalming in ancient Egypt helped push medicine into the male fold.

Male medicine in Egypt emerged in concert with the practice of embalming which, by 2300 BC, had been perfected as a technique. Embalmers were always men. Their practice, which involved the disembowelling of human bodies, led them to a fairly detailed knowledge of anatomy and surgery. They were a smelly, filthy lot, according to Greek historian Herodotus, and were shunned socially, especially by women. They were necrophiliacs; the only women who would hold still for them were dead ones. Because of this practice, high-ranking families retained their female corpses for as long as possible before handing them over to the embalmers, hoping that the advanced processes of decomposition would dissuade the embalmers. A vain hope, we are told.

The embalmers did, however, discover a lot about the human interior. Their findings were written down and used by embalmers and surgeons alike. This knowledge of the inner body became the province of men—and one jealously guarded by them. Male medicine soon stood for knowledge and discovery; women's medicine for superstition.

In line with the growing separation of medicine and religion, medical schools were established at Heliopolis and Sais, Memphis, and later at Alexandria, where both surgeons and embalmers were trained. Sais and Alexandria were the centers of exchange between Greek and Egyptian physicians and surgeons. Moses is said to have studied at Heliopolis and became well-versed in Egyptian medicine, although he continually denounced its practice. The school at Sais specialized in gynecology and obstetrics. The Kahum Papyrus, dated about 2500 BC and thought to have originated at Sais, deals with gynecology as well as veterinary diseases and primarily contains guidance for surgical practice.

Ancient Hebrew society was patriarchal, hierarchical, and authoritarian, permitting one male God and Him alone. The Lord God, Yahveh, was the supreme healer of the sick. The Hebrews knew that deities elsewhere claimed this healing function and that the practice of healing was often in the hands of women, especially in Egypt.

Hebrew leaders would not permit the practice of women healers and, by implication, women priests. Women endured a very low status in their society. The Hebrews had their own story of creation: Adam and Eve and the serpent in the Garden of Eden. The serpent, which, we've been taught symbolizes the knowledge of good and evil, actually symbolized the power and knowledge of women. From time immemorial, in many cultures, the snake was the symbol of healing. For Hebrew society, which denigrated the role of women, the symbolism of crushing the serpent meant the crushing not only of woman's social position, but also of her role in healing. The downfall symbolized the end of the relationship between women and healing.

The ancient Hebrews were a fierce, unforgiving male-oriented society. In their story of creation, their god drove the man and the woman out of the Garden forever. No second chance. Not for them the forgiveness of Ninchursag.

By identifying the practice of healing with their one male god, the Hebrews anticipated the early Christian attitude that sickness was the result of sin and that God alone had authority to heal.

This belief in the one austere male god was in deep contrast to beliefs of the Old Europeans to whom Earth was the Great Mother, and who created maternal images out of water and air divinities. A divinity who nurtures the world with moisture, giving rain—the divine food which metaphorically was understood as mother's milk—naturally became a nurse or a mother figure.

Among the early Greeks the social position of women and their place in medical care was central; the inaccurately reported lowly position of women in classical Greece was greatly exaggerated by the bias of nineteenth-century scholars. But by the time of Hippocrates (460–377 BC), traditional medicine, which used both herb lore and religious ritual and was practiced in the temples primarily by female religious functionaries, was coming into serious disrepute. The male medical schools, particularly the Hippocratic school, formulated hypotheses about the workings of the human body (most of which were wrong) which then became translated into immutable "laws" of nature. These "laws" were not challenged in any rigorous way until the seventeenth and eighteenth centuries.

Medicine was believed to have come of age, to have finally graduated into science, mainly because it was men who were now in charge. Those brave enough to challenge the new precepts were condemned to obscurity. Pliny wrote women healers should be as quiet and inconspicuous as possible so that "after they are dead no one would know they had lived."

Before the fall of Greece, Roman medicine combined religious ritual with practical measures and was handled by women, either in the temples or in their homes.

By the third century BC these women were being cursed and condemned by the intellectuals of the day. Plautus (254–184 BC), Terence (195–159 BC) and Ovid (43 BC–AD 18) all ridiculed women's practice, particularly midwifery, and characterized the midwife, in perhaps the first of all stereotypes, as a superstitious drunk.

After the fall of Greece, the Romans opened their own medical schools based primarily on the teachings of the Hippocratic school. Like the Hebrews, the Romans were patriarchal. Men held the positions of authority and leadership; learning, science, religion and law were all under their control.

Yet women continued to practice healing in the poorer sections of Roman society because the cost of being treated by male doctors was exorbitant. However popular or famous these women healers became through their skills and kindnesses, they functioned strictly as lower-class citizens. Cato haughtily classed them all as abortionists while Galen (AD 129–201) referred to traditional medicine as "old wives' tales and Egyptian quackeries." These male attitudes are hardly surprising when one considers that the women's practice was at variance with the male medical theory and practice of the day; even more important, it was a challenge to patriarchal ideology.

The conversion of the Roman empire to Christianity hardened attitudes toward women and women healers. Roman gods were replaced by one all-powerful male God whose duties included healing, and who delegated the role of healing to His chosen successors—males.

The early Christian church of Rome found itself confronted by midwives and women healers who represented an open challenge to the church's views on sickness and disease as well as on the role and position of women in society.

It taught that one was sick according to God's will; sickness was the result of sin. Healing was a matter of forgiveness. Anyone who thought otherwise and sought relief from pain by means other than prayer was condemned. And any attempt to cure was certain evidence of paganism or devilish inspiration or both.

Healing, then, became sorcery, and women healers were the servants of demons. While belief in Satan was as important an aspect of the Christian religion as was belief in God, belief in other peoples' demons was denounced as paganism. And to be pagan was to be criminal. As Christianity spread throughout Europe, old laws were revised to deal with this new and terrifying consideration. So those who went to the women healers went in secret and with fear in their hearts.

Then, as now, there were those arrogant enough to speak for God. Medicine, they said, was a sinful act and the practice of healing—especially if it succeeded—"could only be by the help of devils and whoever sought to do anything, even good, by such means must be God's enemy." The association between women, healing, sorcery, and the Devil became enshrined in canon and civil law. Translations of the period have changed original meanings of words from *female healers* to incorrectly read *witches* and *sorceresses*.

In time the church announced to the known world the true reason for all of women's failings. Beginning about the twelfth century, Christian theologians proclaimed that women suffered from a spiritual deficiency which left them helpless to withstand temptation by the Devil. Here was possibly the greatest insult to date. Women couldn't even be evil on their own; they must first be subjected to a male authority. The Devil, like God, was always conceptualized in masculine form.

Now the study of medicine was primarily concerned with

the study of theology and the new university-trained physicians were not allowed to practice without first calling a priest to aid and advise them. Nor were they allowed to treat a patient who refused confession. The doctors' practice consisted largely of bleedings and cuppings (drawing blood by cutting the skin and applying a cupping glass), christianized incantations (prayer), and astrology.

Practical experience was absent in their training, so what practical knowledge they had was derived largely from old wives, or wise women. In the thirteenth century, for example, one professor at Oxford rode forty miles to get a prescription from an old woman who cured jaundice with the cooked juice of plantain. And in 1527 Paracelsus burned his medical texts, confessing that "he had learned from the sorceress all he knew."

By the seventeenth century, the church announced it knew what was wrong with women. Not only were they open to the temptations of sensuality, they were also illogical and irrational; there was something wrong with their brains and their bodies. Women had things inside them—strange organs—that made them crazy and sinful.

In one respect, the early church was right; evil *was* all around. It was the most terrible of evils, conjured up by that strange alchemy of ignorance, superstition, pride, hatred, jealousy. And it ignited into a holocaust—the persecution of women on charges of witchcraft.

It had been a long time smoldering. Yet even those terrible bloodbaths did not eliminate woman's role as healer; the demands and needs of the poor kept her going. The prime motivation of these persecutions was not only to eliminate women in healing. The period of these tortures, beginning in Europe in the fourteenth century and ending in England in the seventeenth century, was too long and too complex to support such a simplistic solution.

The issue was far broader. It was a concerted attempt to usurp woman's place in the natural world. Fed by clerical thunderings, the fires burned hot as living women were bound to the stake—wise women, "old wives," who had preserved traditional skills and knowledge down through time.

The witchcraft persecutions established a point in history at which attitudes toward women and toward healing were enshrined in official legislation. For the first time, physicians saw themselves as members of a closed profession and demanded protection so that a monopoly of the male ascendancy could be guaranteed and preserved.

Finally, after centuries of conflict and cunning, woman was dethroned. By authority of the penis, medicine was the province of males. Control of the essence of womanhood—her sexual and reproductive life—was the great prize.

By the beginning of the nineteenth century medicine was firmly in the hands of males, and the Great Cut was about to begin. Women still had those strange organs inside them that made them crazy. Soon it would be clear that women would be greatly improved if these things were cut out.

The doctors of those days were far more than businessmen weighing female physiology against cash flow. By their own definition they were men of science, working in a cultural framework that equated science with goodness and morality. They saw themselves as moral reformers.

According to Darwin's theory of evolution, man had evolved from lower, or less complex, forms of life to his present exalted status. The gentlemen of medicine didn't take this to mean *mankind*, which was Darwin's meaning, but man as in male vs. female. A monumental body of research involving measurements of brain weights, head sizes, and facial proportions "proved" that WASPS (white, Anglo-Saxon Protestants) were in first place, followed by Northern Europeans, Slavs, Jews, Italians, and so on. Blacks were so far down as to be almost unrecognizable. Where was woman? Certainly not up there with her husband. She was at the level of the black, which was nowhere at all.

Now doctors agreed that even the ancient Greeks knew about the uterus and ovaries from poking about in dead bodies.

Women had these organs, men did not. It was only logical, the old Greeks had proved, that hysteria was caused by some purely female organ. So the word *hysteria* or "suffering caused by the uterus" began its career with the Greek word *hysterikos*. The trouble with women was the fault of their specialized body parts.

A woman's uterus and ovaries were blamed for an improbable array of female disorders ranging from headaches to sore throats and indigestion. Everything was blamed on the ovaries or "a disease of the womb." Even tuberculosis in women was traced to their ovaries. When men got TB, however, doctors sought some environmental factor to explain the disease. In women, it was caused by their sexual systems.

Logically enough, the next step was treatment for all of these pernicious wombs and ovaries. Backaches, irritability, indigestion, and liver malfunction could provoke a medical assault on the female sexual organs. Treatment included manual investigation, leeching, injections, and cauterization. Leeches were placed directly on the vulva or the cervix, although doctors were cautioned to be sure to count the animals as they dropped off full of blood. Adventurous leeches sometimes advanced into the cervical canal itself. One gynecologist wrote: "I think I have scarcely ever seen more acute pain than that experienced by several of my patients under these circumstances."

Injections, made directly into the womb, included water, milk and water, linseed tea, and "decoction of marshmallow . . . tepid or cold."

One of the most severe treatments was cauterization, performed by the application of nitrate of silver or, in cases of more severe infection, the far stronger hydrate of potassa. Even more painful was the burning of the cervix, called actual cautery, by a white-hot iron instrument. No anesthetic was used except for a little opium or alcohol.

In 1846 a demonstration occurred at the Massachusetts General Hospital which we now know had great import for women. Gone were the leeches and cautery after surgeon John Collins Warren and dentist W. T. G. Morton anesthetized Gilbert Abbott, and removed a neck tumor.

With the advent of anesthesiology, doctors could *really* take care of women's problems: they could cut them out! And cut they did. According to W. H. R. Rivers' 1924 book, *Medicine, Magic and Religion,* medical indications for surgery included: ". . . troublesomeness, eating like a ploughman, masturbation, attempted suicide, erotic tendencies, persecution mania, simple cussedness, and dysmenorrhea (painful menstruation). Most apparent in the enormous variety of symptoms doctors took to indicate castration was a strong current of sexual appetiveness on the part of women."

Untold thousands of uteruses and ovaries were excised. A pioneer in the field was Dr. Robert Battey, an ambitious surgeon from Rome, Georgia, who argued in the 1870s that removal of the ovaries would bring women a salutary change of life. His postoperative patients, he said, were "tractable, orderly, industrious and cleanly." His extensive experience, using women as guinea pigs, is said to have greatly advanced abdominal surgery techniques.

Soon most doctors jumped into the Ovary Arena, reasoning that since the ovaries controlled the personality, they must be responsible for any psychological disorders. Conversely, psychological disorders were a sure sign of ovarian disease. A woman relieved of her ovaries would be a *better* woman. One 1893 enthusiast of the operation, a man, said that "patients are improved, some of them cured . . . the moral sense of the patient is elevated . . ."

Many patients were brought in by their husbands who complained of their wives' unruly or lustful behavior. Doctors wrote that women, troublesome but still sane enough to recognize their problems, often "come to us pleading to have their ovaries removed." If the woman subsequently became a placid creature, content with her domestic functions, cried a lot but expected nothing else out of life, the operation was considered a huge success. She was spayed.

By the late nineteenth and early twentieth centuries, the medical profession was supported by one common thought: femininity was a disease. It was a woman's normal state to be sick. This was decreed as a physiological fact, not just an empirical observation. Medicine had officially discovered what the early church had decreed centuries ago—females have bad things inside of them. Women accepted the dogma that they were in desperate need of the surgeons' scalpels. And the scalpels of salvation swung into play.

A few feminists placed much of the blame on doctors' financial interests. Mary Livermore spoke against "the monstrous assumption that woman is a natural invalid," and denounced the "unclean army of 'gynecologists' who seem desirous to convince women that they possess but one set of organs—and that these are always diseased."

Dr. Mary Putnam said: ". . . it is in the increased attention paid to women, and especially in their new function as lucrative patients, scarcely imagined a hundred years ago, that we find explanation for much of the ill-health among women, freshly discovered today . . ."

Women were forbidden to enjoy sex, being sternly warned against any "spasmodic convulsion" during intercourse lest it interfere with conception. Like the church of old, doctors feared that woman's "insatiable lust," once awakened, would turn out to be uncontrollable. Terrible stories were told of women destroyed by their cravings. One doctor said he had discovered a case of "virgin nymphomania." Another, the twenty-five-year-old British physician, Robert Brudenell Carter, observed: ". . . I have seen young married women of the middle class of society reduced by the constant use of the speculum to the mental and moral condition of prostitutes; seeking to give themselves the same indulgence by the practice of solitary vice; and asking every medical practitioner to institute an examination of the sexual organs." Young Dr. Carter was much admired in spite of the contempt for women expressed in his statement.

Reproduction was woman's grand purpose in life. At puberty, girls were to take a great deal of bed rest to help focus their energies on regulating their periods, and were warned that too much reading or intellectual stimulation in the fragile stage of adolescence would result in permanent damage to their reproductive organs. Doctors forbade the reading of romantic novels as "one of the greatest causes of uterine disease in young women."

Some of the finest minds of the day preached that higher education would cause women's uteruses to atrophy. Dr. Edward H. Clarke, a Harvard professor, authored the curiously titled *Sex in Education or a Fair Chance for the Girls,* at the height of the pressure for coeducation at Harvard. Considered the great uterine manifesto of the ninteenth century, the book went through seventeen editions in just a few years.

Dr. S. Weir Mitchell, a Philadelphia physician, argued that women were unfit to use their minds because of disqualifications existing in their physiological life, their "female organs." Now considered the greatest pioneer in the development of the expert-to-woman relationship, Dr. Mitchell perfected the technique of healing by command. He was *the* doctor for hundreds of loyal women patients, earning, at the height of his career in the 1880s, over $60,000 a year (over $695,000 in today's dollars). His treatments were flashy: surgical, electrical, hydropathic, mesmeric, chemical. None of them seemed to do anybody any real good, but it didn't matter. The women loved him.

His famous rest cure was extremely popular. The woman undergoing this cure was isolated and subjected to sensory deprivation, with one exception, for six weeks. She was made to lie on her back in a dimly lit room. She was not permitted to read. If Dr. Mitchell considered her case severe, she was not even permitted to rise to urinate. She could have no visitors, see no males; she could only see a nurse and Dr. Mitchell himself. The one exception to sensory deprivation was a long, sensual massage every day.

In Dr. Mitchell's battle against the uterus, he frequently called into play another organ, the phallus, penetrating a recalcitrant patient's will with the force of his masculinity. The so-called "male force" had long been recognized in medicine. Earlier treatments had already recognized the need for direct male penetration to set females on the right track. Nineteenth-century doctors expected women to spread their legs to admit leeches, cautery, scalpel, or whatever the physician chose to insert. And the so-called "final argument" against women doctors was that they could not "obtain the needed control over those of their own sex." Possession of a penis meant control over the female patient and only a male could command the total submissiveness that constituted the cure. In Dr. Mitchell's case, if a patient failed to recover at the end of her rest cure, he would threaten to take off his trousers and climb into bed with her, actually removing his clothing until the patient leapt out of bed in a fury.

In the 1890s, Charlotte Perkins Gilman, who had observed that her sickness vanished when she was away from her home, husband, and child and returned as soon as she came back to them, borrowed one hundred dollars from a friend of her mother's for the trip to Philadelphia and Mitchell's treatment.

Being a writer, Gilman methodically wrote out a complete history of her case. Mitchell dismissed her prepared history as evidence of "self-conceit," stating that he did not want information from his patients, he wanted "complete obedience."

She gritted her teeth, underwent the cure, then returned home with the following directions from Dr. Mitchell:

"Live as domestic a life as possible. Have your child with you at all times. [If she even dressed the baby it left her shaking and crying.] Lie down for an hour after each meal. Have but two hours intellectual life a day. And never touch pen, brush or pencil as long as you live."

For some months she attempted to follow the doctor's orders. She almost lost her mind. "The mental agony grew so unbearable that I would sit blankly moving my head from side to side. I would crawl into remote closets and under beds—to hide from the grinding pressure of that distress."

Fortunately for Charlotte Gilman, she enjoyed a "moment of clear vision," and realized she did not want to be a wife. She wanted to be a writer and an activist (two very suspect occupations).

155

She divorced both her husband and S. Weir Mitchell, took off for California with her baby, her pen, her brush, and her pencil. Three years later she wrote *The Yellow Wallpaper*, a chilling and realistic account of descent into madness.

After a long life of accomplishments, she wrote that if her story had any influence on S. Weir Mitchell's method of treatment, "I have not lived in vain."

Charlotte Perkins Gilman figured out her predicament for herself. She finally understood what was happening to her. Thousands of other women found themselves in a new position of subservience to the male medical profession with no other sources for information or counsel.

The woman who felt sick or tired or discouraged or depressed would no longer seek help from a friend or a female healer. She went, instead, to a male physician, who knew that women by nature were weak, dependent, and diseased. Doctors had secured their victory over the female healer with "scientific" evidence that woman's essential nature was to be sick. "She's not a well woman, you know," was the pass-phrase of the day.

And women certainly did have problems, over and above their physicians. In the nineteenth century, a married woman could expect to face the risk of childbirth repeatedly through her fertile years. After each birth, she could well suffer from any number of gynecological complications which would either kill her or be with her the rest of her life. In 1915, the first year for which national figures are available, sixty-one women died for every ten thousand live babies born, compared to two per ten thousand today.

In addition, there were thousands of women whose uteruses and ovaries had been cut out and who, all unwittingly, suffered terribly from hormone deprivation—not a natural diminuendo, but the abrupt, punishing kind brought on by the scalpel.

Then a new kind of doctor appeared on the scene—the psychoanalyst. At first it was a contest, with both factions struggling for possession of woman as patient. Freud legiti-mized a doctor-patient relationship based on talking, not cut-ting, although he frequently turned his own patients over to the surgeons, notably Wilhelm Fliess, the nose and throat phy-sician who was his closest friend between 1894 and 1900, the years Freud was formulating his theories. Fleiss held the strange belief that the nose and the sexual organs were intimately con-nected and that sexual problems could be cured through nasal surgery. Freud's therapy urged the patient to confess her re-sentments and rebelliousness and then, at last, accept her role as a *true woman*. He deduced that women are masochistic by nature and crave what he called "the lust of pain," a dogma first voiced by him in a little known 1924 paper entitled *The Economic Problem in Masochism*. In this paper Freud unveiled his psychoanalytic theory that masochism in women is the pre-ferred state, an expression of sexual maturity or, in his own terms, "the final genital stage obtaining from the situation characteristic of womanhood, namely, the passive part in co-itus and the act of giving birth."

What Freud said was that woman is the helpless, passive receptor, rather than the originator, of life. Men and sex *hap-pen* to her; children *happen* to her. At that time, and in many ways, this was true. Through the centuries woman had been maneuvered into a position of *object*. She was to take no plea-sure in sex. She was to have no orgasm. She was to take no active part in the birth of her children. She was to let someone take out her uterus and ovaries as soon as her childbearing was done.

After physicians and psychoanalysts decided to coexist (they had to for neither faction was going away), doctors sent their complaining postsurgical patients over for sessions on the couch. Obviously, if a woman complained that she was horribly de-pressed, listless, cared no longer about her husband, hardly cared whether she lived or died, she had to be crazy. For cer-tainly she *should* be far better off without her uterus and ova-ries.

And women went to the surgeons, and thought they were crazy, and many of them committed suicide, or were confined to mental institutions. Today, women don't go to mental institutions, for the most part, because supplemental hormones are available. But they're still looked at doubtfully when they complain of problems that supplemental hormones don't take care of.

For well over a century, women have relinquished their insides with scarcely a question. Many of them continue to do so because there are far too many physicians who feel that women would be a lot better off without "that whole mess."

Chapter Ten

HOW TO AVOID HYSTERECTOMY AND HOW TO GET HELP IF YOU'VE HAD ONE

Because the female genitals are, for the most part, hidden, women have traditionally felt they needed someone else to validate that the organs were there at all—and that they were all right or all wrong.

For this validation, women turn to gynecologists, most of whom believe that hysterectomy is a benevolent surgery, that it is done solely to "remove disease."

What about *curing* the disease instead of cutting everything out?

Other physicians claim, relative to libido, that enjoyment of sex is purely a mental phenomenon and is in no way dependent on whether the uterus and ovaries are present; that these organs have only to do with pregnancy and nothing at all to do with sexual desire and gratification. How far can members of the medical profession who make questionable statements like this be trusted? How far can the medical profession itself be trusted? When doctors passed out Valium by the carload, for example, they did not reveal that the side effects were anxiety, stress, muscle tension, suicidal depression—the very symptoms for which they were prescribing the drug!

The ability to function sexually is an important part of life. When dysfunction occurs, the negative effects on a woman's emotional life are widespread and significant.

Hysterectomy is a surgery that literally alters a woman, cutting major vessels and arteries that flow to the hormone centers of the body and cutting through or removing sensory pathways. Because of its effect on these centers and pathways, it changes the way a woman thinks about herself and how she interacts with others. It changes surrounding muscle structures. It cruelly affects sexual desire, turning many women into what one aware doctor calls "sexual mutes." Some women suffer depression, thoughts of suicide, and total frigidity while others develop a genital anesthesia.

When a woman undergoes a needless hysterectomy, the emotional aspects are considerable. She is totally powerless to reverse the procedure, to go back in time, to recover or re-grow her lost organs. She is baffled by unwelcome changes in herself for which she can find no answers. She suffers. Those around her suffer. Her relationships change. She has lost a lot. Studies on the long-term effects of unnecessary surgery done on women are frightening. The population of women abounds with tragedies—heartbreaking aftermaths of overanxious scalpels.

Is it possible for a woman to avoid hysterectomy? Can a woman who has already undergone hysterectomy get help for her hormonal and sexual problems?

The answer to both questions is a resounding *yes*.

How to Avoid a Hysterectomy

The first and most obvious way is simply not to have the surgery. One should not be so eager to surrender one's uterus and ovaries to the scalpel but should take the time and trouble to choose a physician who will be honest about one's true condition and one's options. Obviously, judgment and good sense are required on the part of both patient and physician, for there are a few cases where such avoidance could be a terrible—and lethal—mistake.

It *is* possible for a woman to avoid some of the conditions that lead to hysterectomy. The use of modern birth control pills (whose forerunners were the subject of much bad publicity due to cases of pulmonary embolism) has been found to prevent many of the problems associated with menstrual irregularity, often a harbinger of or prelude to severe adenomatous hyperplasia, an endometrial condition which can be the same as early carcinoma of the endometrium. The rate of ovarian cancer has also been found to be much lower in women who take birth control pills.

The use of ultrasound and laparoscopy can also reduce the incidence of hysterectomy by informing the physician of a woman's condition without resorting to major surgery. Ultrasound is used to check changes in the size of the ovaries. In the case of uterine enlargement where the physician can't be sure if the ovaries are involved, ultrasound will reveal any enlargements.

Laparoscopy, done under local anesthesia, involves making a tiny slit in the woman's abdomen, inserting the laparoscope and viewing what's going on inside. It is especially helpful in determining the cause of pelvic pain and ovarian enlargement. In many cases the physician, by knowing in advance what a woman's condition is, can provide medical treatment instead of hysterectomy.

Women whose lifestyles include a variety of sexual partners can avoid some of the conditions that lead to hysterectomy by protecting themselves from possible infections. Thousands of hysterectomies are done for chronic and recurrent PID (Pelvic Inflammatory Disease), a condition in which the tubes and ovaries have severely deteriorated because of recurring infection.

Abortion centers play a role in helping women avoid hysterectomy. These centers provide medically qualified people to handle the procedure in a clinical atmosphere. Before abortion was legalized, untold numbers of women went to back-room, unskilled operators and too frequently emerged with their insides so torn up—or developed such severe infections due to dirty operating conditions—that total hysterectomy was mandatory to save their lives.

Perhaps most important, a woman should try very hard to find a doctor who is interested in helping her *avoid* surgery. Internists, for example, may suggest nonsurgical alternatives not offered by ob/gyns and general surgeons. Such doctors are sometimes called conservative because they don't immediately resort to the knife unless they believe it is absolutely necessary to do so.

Another option is holistic medicine, a catchall phrase for a variety of alternative healing forms including nutrition, exercise, visualization, meditation, acupuncture, chiropractic, naturopathic, homeopathic, herbal and nutritional therapies, to name a few. Holistic health, meaning *whole body health,* is an active state of health, a unity of mind, body, and spirit; not the absence of disease but rather a state of vibrant well being. Medicine, as such, is a small part of holistic health. There has been some reluctance on the part of conventional medicine to acknowledge holistic procedures, but it is now advocated by the surgeon general of the United States and practiced by Walter Reed Hospital.

Sarah J., a dealer in antiques, had been having rather heavy periods for several years. Her regular physician didn't think the symptoms were too important.

A friend told her she should be alarmed about the bleeding, so Sarah visited a gynecologist who, after doing a pelvic exam, asked if she had seen her family physician within the last six months. She told him that she had.

"Then it's almost certain you have cancer," the gynecologist said. "You have a growth in your uterus and if it's as obvious as it is now, and you saw your regular doctor six months ago, it's grown too rapidly to be anything but malignant."

He summoned his office nurse to make an appointment for surgery but was told no surgical suites were immediately available. As Sarah was leaving, in a state of shock and fear, the nurse caught her. "You're in luck! The hospital just called back. There's been a cancellation and we can get you in for surgery tomorrow. Go home and pack a bag, then get right over there."

Sarah made it home, trembling with fright. Then her pragmatic nature took over and she thought that just maybe she'd been hustled a little too fast. She decided to get a second opinion. A friend recommended another gynecologist. He also told her she had a growth and wanted to operate immediately. She went to yet a third gynecologist who, as did the other two, declared he should do an immediate removal of uterus and both ovaries.

Just before finally committing herself for surgery, she heard about a doctor who practiced holistic medicine. She saw him and was delighted when he said she didn't need surgery, that he could treat her medically. He was a naturopath. Under his care, the heavy bleeding stopped and she felt good, more energetic than ever before. She said the only problem was that after intercourse she bled just a little. She was afraid that her lover, who subsequently became her husband, "wouldn't be able to handle that."

She said: "I was really embarrassed about the post-coital bleeding and I did a very stupid thing. I stopped seeing the holistic man and shopped around for a gynecologist with whom I felt comfortable."

She found him. This fourth gynecologist told her it would be better to get "completely cleaned out, particularly since you don't want children." The surgery was done.

"Now I had a real problem," she said. "My whole sex life was in shambles. After a couple of years with no improvement, the doctor who did the hysterectomy said he could do a tightening of the vagina which would make sex enjoyable for me again. I had it done but it was really a mistake. It just made sex totally uncomfortable as well as unfulfilling. As for desire, I haven't felt any since before the hysterectomy, which was done five years ago."

Women must never forget that, except in extremely rare cases, hysterectomy is an elective procedure. This means *a woman can choose whether or not to have it done.* A woman's body belongs to herself. It does not belong to her husband, lover, children, or doctor. Although she may welcome an interested person with whom to discuss the pros and cons, she must in the end make her own decision. Especially she should make her own decision about retaining her ovaries, remembering that they protect her through the continued production of estrogen, progesterone, and androgens.

Women can take heart that there are some doctors—admittedly few as yet—who are sensitive to the special problems women face.

Such a doctor is Vicki Georges Hufnagel, a prominent gynecologist who practices in West Los Angeles. A new pioneer in women's medicine, Dr. Hufnagel is responsible for research and discovery of some of the best state of the art techniques presently available, including Female Reconstructive Surgery and the various uses of the ultrasound machine.

Dr. Hufnagel has spent the past five years pioneering alternative procedures to hysterectomy and has developed what is called Female Reconstructive Surgery (FRS), a combination of techniques that enable a woman to maintain her sexual organs by treating and curing symptoms. Common symptoms that trigger a doctor to prescribe hysterectomy, Dr. Hufnagel says, are bleeding between periods, fibroid tumors, cramps, abnormal hormonal function, and scarification of earlier infections or operations, which can cause some or all of the foregoing.

Figures from the U.S. Department of Health and Human Resources support Dr. Hufnagel's claim that only 4.7 percent of hysterectomies performed in the United States today are necessary surgeries.

"The medical profession, both male and female, has been taught for the past eighty years that hysterectomies are THE solution to everything from fibroid tumors, cramps and heavy bleeding," she says. "Doctors who do this are practicing medicine by looking in the rearview mirror. Otherwise, why is a ninety-year-old procedure the most commonly performed surgery? Nothing else devised in the 1890s is used today."

Dr. Hufnagel says that millions of women have already lost their uteruses, and that many more millions will yet lose their uteruses needlessly unless there is a fundamental change in medicine. She treats all of the conditions that usually indicate hysterectomy by conservative medical methods including surgery—but without hysterectomy. As an example, for prolapse of the uterus, she has developed what is called the Hufnagel Procedure for resuspending the pelvic organs. Using the latest microsurgery, laser and ultrasound techniques, she removes scars and adhesions from prior surgery, infection and/or endometriosis, along with removing fibroid tumors. She also reconnects fallopian tubes after sterilization. She reports that many women suffer from pain and abnormal menstrual cycles following sterilization and that their symptoms disappear after reconstructive surgery.

Hysterectomy, she says, is easier to do from a surgical standpoint than Female Reconstructive Surgery (FRS), but is a "real butchery" operation. She declares that the only time a hysterectomy is truly necessary is in the case of cancer, obstetrical catastrophe or tuberculosis. The former two are rare and the latter is seldom seen in industrialized countries.

"Hysterectomy involves a high rate of complications," she asserts. "Not only is it a major operation, with all the risks *that* entails, but there are common complications such as hematomas, profuse bleeding, infection, bladder problems, urinary retention, kidney infection, and many more. The operation creates false menopause, accelerates aging, and increases psychological and hormonal stresses."

She says that depression following hysterectomy is not feminine hysteria, as so many claim, but rather has a very real chemical cause, adding that "it's the lack of feminine hormone feedback in the pituitary gland that's to blame. For years, doctors have put women on lithium and Valium, which are psychoactive drugs, for mood swings or anxiety following hysterectomy. But the stress, distress, and emotional crises are caused by hormonal abnormalities, not the psyche."

Dr. Hufnagel has unequivocally shown that fibroid tumors never equal hysterectomy, although that's the most common excuse for the operation. Most fibroids grow inside the walls of the uterus, she says, and they can be removed without sacrificing the uterus or the ovaries. Although some other surgeons perform tumor removal on a limited number of tumors, Dr. Hufnagel has removed as many as 138 tumors during an eight-hour surgery.

During her five years of performing FRS, Dr. Hufnagel has achieved 100 percent success. Most of her patients, who come from all over the world, are out of the hospital in three to four days, their childbearing capabilities, sexual desire and hormonal flows intact. The simple, almost bloodless procedure is beyond conventional myomectomy, which is why she has named it Female Reconstructive Surgery.

Her successes include the removal of tumors that had been declared "inoperable" by other surgeons. One young woman had been cut open twice, only to be told that her tumor was inoperable because of its size and placement. The third time she was opened up, Dr. Hufnagel removed a tumor the size of a football and did the necessary repair work, leaving the patient's perfectly good female organs intact.

One thirty-year-old woman, whose fibroid was as large as a basketball, went to twenty-two physicians, all of whom told her she must have an immediate hysterectomy. Then she heard about Dr. Hufnagel. Using an epidural anesthesia so that the patient was awake the entire time, Dr. Hufnagel removed the tumor and reconstructed the uterus. This woman, who normally would have been castrated, now has the opportunity to have the children she desperately wants.

No matter the size of the tumor or the number of tumors, they can usually be removed by Dr. Hufnagel's technique without damaging the uterus. She says size doesn't matter but what *is* important is the location of the tumor or tumors and which blood vessels are involved. Less than .02 percent of fibroids are malignant, Dr. Hufnagel says, adding that these tumors probably do not *grow* into cancer; the seed of the cancer is already there.

Although doctors in the United States are beginning to learn about Dr. Hufnagel's techniques for performing FRS as an alternative to hysterectomy, she says it's still an uphill battle, simply because it's easier for surgeons to chop something out during a forty-five-minute surgery rather than spend the four to eight hours that FRS requires. And, too, there is always resistance to change.

Consulting a Physician

It is a good idea to take notes or, if the doctor has no objection, to tape the conversation. On the average, patients remember only about 10 percent of what doctors tell them. This forgetfulness is a result of a certain amount of fear and stress involved in the patient-physician relationship.

Don't be afraid to insult your physician with questions. Increased knowledge will decrease your anxieties. Don't be cowed by a holier-than-thou attitude, or a refusal to answer your questions. You don't need a doctor like this. Fire him or her and find another.

If your doctor recommends a hysterectomy, consult at least *four* others. One other is not enough. Unfortunately, even with second—and third—opinions, the hysterectomy rate is on the rise. Most doctors stick together. It is a tradition taught them in medical school and, as in any other business, what's good for one is good for all. Most of the women interviewed for this book got second and even third opinions and were still operated on. Remember: hysterectomy is big business and an awful lot of doctors would have to take down their shingles if no woman bought hysterectomy anymore.

Ask each doctor the following ten questions:

1. *How many hysterectomies have you performed over what period of time?*
   If he's performed a lot, get away from him. That means he likes them and makes his living doing them. You can be sure he'll recommend one for you.
2. *What, in your opinion, are the medical indications for hysterectomy?*

If he tells you the only real indication for hysterectomy is uterine cancer, you'll know he's not knife-happy.

3. *How long will you treat a condition before deciding that surgery is unavoidable?*
If he tells you it is customary for him to treat a condition for several years—exclusive of known uterine cancer—you've probably got yourself a pretty good doctor.

4. *What are some of the treatments you advise?*
If he tells you he would do a myomectomy to remove troublesome fibroid tumors rather than a hysterectomy, that's a good sign. Other positive indications are his regular testing of blood levels of your hormones to keep them at normal levels; drawing of estrogen and progesterone levels, called an FSH-LH, every six months; and a study called a QCT, which studies the bones in your spine to see if you are developing osteoporosis. He should also be able to counsel you in nutrition and holistic health approaches.

5. *Do you admit that many women suffer severe sexual problems following hysterectomy?*
If he says he knows this is true, he is an aware, caring physician.

6. *How do you feel about leaving the ovaries in should I need to have my uterus removed?*
If he says he would never remove the ovaries unless they were cancerous, he's good.

7. *Are you willing to work with a patient who will do almost anything to avoid hysterectomy?*
He should say yes without reservation.

8. *Do you prescribe endocrine therapy following hysterectomy?*
Again, he should say yes without reservation.

9. *Do you mind if I get a third and even a fourth opinion?*
He should encourage you to do this. However, if *he* suggests the doctors you should consult, you should be aware of the implications this presents.

10. *Do you provide or recommend post-hysterectomy sexual counseling?*

If he either provides or recommends post-hysterectomy counseling, he's advanced enough to realize that many women suffer severe sexual problems following this kind of surgery. If, however, he starts talking about psychological problems, about your feeling less of a woman, about your marital adjustment, and so forth, he's simply singing the same old song that's been on the Medical Hit and Miss Parade for years. And if he talks about your perception of your femininity, run, don't walk, to the nearest exit.

If your doctor is a responsive, understanding person, level with him. Talk about yourself. Many women complain: "Most of the doctors won't even listen to me." If you don't feel that your doctor is answering your questions satisfactorily, get another doctor.

If you have a gynecologist whom you can really talk to, who sees and understands you as a woman, as a human being—not just as figures on a billing record—treasure him or her forever.

If, for whatever reason, you do need to have your uterus removed, be extremely careful you don't go to a doctor who will announce after the operation: "Well, as long as I was in there, I took out the tubes, and to save you another operation later, I took out the ovaries. And since I was in there anyway I took out the appendix." Before surgery request that your doctor sign a statement that he will not remove your ovaries without your full knowledge and consent.

Doctors do a lot of things without a woman's consent. I've been told of one who decides whether a woman's clitoris is in the wrong place for sexual satisfaction, and then moves it to what he considers the right place. He has reportedly performed thousands of these moving jobs, most of them without the patient's consent because he does it during the course of another surgery!

There is another salient point to remember. Whenever doctors go out on strike, the mortality rate promptly drops. It happened in Saskatchewan in 1968. It happened in Los Angeles in 1974; the mortality rate dropped by 18 percent. In Columbia, South America, the doctors went out on strike and the mortality rate dropped by 37 percent. In Israel, during an eighty-seven-day strike, the mortality rate dropped by 50 percent.

No matter how handsome he looks in his houndstooth blazer, your doctor is not a god. He doesn't always know best. But he *can* learn a lot from you, if he's smart enough to know it. Help him help you.

Remember: the only thing a male doctor knows about being a woman he knows by hearsay.

When Hysterectomy Is Called For

If after consultation and deliberation a woman has made the decision for hysterectomy, it would be well for her, both before and after surgery, to eat a diet high in protein, vitamins, and minerals to replenish the serious losses of body nutrients that surgery causes. She may also wish to take supplements of Vitamins A, B, C, and D as well as zinc and iron.

Before entering the hospital, she should find out the hospital's policies. One woman discovered that her lesbian partner was excluded from the intensive care unit because, being neither "family" nor spouse, she had no "legitimate" claim.

The New Our Bodies, Ourselves advises that once hospitalized, a woman should:

1. Know the name of the one doctor in charge of her case.
2. Whenever tests or X-rays are proposed, ask why. Such technology vastly increases overall hospital cost, further depersonalizes care, and is often applied inappropriately.
3. If possible, establish rapport with the nursing staff. Nurses are the true coordinators of one's total care and keep their own records, which are separate from those

of the doctor. Their judgments can influence an entire course of care.

4. Try to get *out* of the hospital as soon as possible. There are nearly continuous outbreaks of infection in most hospitals which are increasingly resistant to antibiotic treatments.

5. Choose local anesthesia, if at all possible, rather than general anesthesia. Locals enable a patient to recover more quickly and don't carry the same risk of death.

6. Discover what medicines have been prescribed and by whom, for what purpose, and how often they are to be taken. Ask nurses which medications they are giving her; then try to keep a record of them and cross-check with her physician. Resist routine tranquilizers and sleeping pills. (Try milk at bedtime instead of juice because milk contains L-tryptophan, a natural relaxant.)

7. Ask friends to bring good food daily. Hospital food is frequently not nutritious.

8. Be supplied with bottled spring water. In some areas of the country hospital water has been shown to be contaminated by bacteria.

9. Upon leaving the hospital, request a copy of your records. They may be useful in the future and some hospitals destroy records after a short period of time.

Help for the Post-Hysterectomy Woman

Women who have already undergone the surgery and find themselves suffering from any or all of the post-hysterectomy symptoms *can* obtain help if they understand their condition and what has brought it about.

Recent medical studies have shown what has long been suspected by many women—that estrogen deficiency has an important role in depression brought on by ovary removal. When both ovaries have been taken out, the ovarian function stops abruptly, resulting in serious hormonal changes that are responsible for a variety of clinical manifestations including insomnia, hot flashes, osteoporosis, depression, and sexual dysfunction. Almost every system in a woman undergoes change after ovarian removal. Atrophic changes in the vagina may make sexual relations uncomfortable; atrophic changes in the bladder and sphincter mechanisms can cause such urinary symptoms as increased frequency and stress incontinence. Lipid concentration alterations have been shown to cause increased cardiovascular complications. Many of these conditions can be improved by hormone therapy.

Regarding estrogen therapy, women whose uteruses have been removed can take estrogen safely. Estrogen therapy should be accompanied by some form or exercise—walking is excellent—and elimination of smoking and drinking alcoholic beverages. A woman who still has her uterus is usually given synthetic progesterone along with estrogen to avoid stimulation of the lining of the uterus and the possible risk of cancer.

Some women swear by pellet implantation (a minor procedure done in the doctor's office) for hormone therapy. Many others take hormones in the form of tablets. Still others seem to derive no benefit from oral hormones and rely on shots every three or four weeks. Doctors feel that some women's systems—a fault, perhaps, in the breakdown between ingestion and metabolism—prevent any benefit from oral doses. These women are helped by intramuscular shots that are immediately absorbed into the blood stream.

Samantha S. is a forty-five-year-old owner of a real estate agency. She had always felt she was oversexed, a belief reinforced by her ex-husband. "Which is why he's my ex," she laughed.

She and her present husband had been married for seven years when her doctor found fibroid tumors. They weren't giving her any trouble, but, because of her age, he strongly recommended a hysterectomy and oophorectomy. When a second doctor advised the same procedure, she returned to her regular gynecologist and had the surgery performed. "I wasn't going to wait around until I got cancer like he said was possible."

Samantha, an ardent journal keeper, shared the following excerpt:

April 22—It is now 12 noon. I had a shot at about 11:15 this a.m. When I woke up this a.m. I couldn't stand to look at Sam [her husband], actively disliked him as I always do when I need my hormone shot. My mind was fuzzy, I couldn't think straight, every bone in my body ached. I felt extremely depressed as if the slightest emotional pressure or a wrong look from anybody would set me to suicide. I didn't think it had been that long since I'd had my last shot so I called the nurse who told me it had been over three weeks.

I've learned not to wait and try to bull it out. Time goes so rapidly I find it hard to believe it had already been that long. Experience has shown me that if I wait, life is simply not worth living for me or anyone around me. So I ran out and got shot.

Now, just within the last five minutes, I feel as if a whole bunch of cobwebs have been wiped from my brain. I can think quite clearly and my energy is returning.

Can't believe the difference one tiny shot makes. The nurse told me today that each month after she gets her shot she thinks, oh, well, this is probably all in my head and I will just rise above it. But it never works. She agrees with me that she can understand how women commit suicide when they're deprived of hormones. It's NO JOKE! Gad, how I hate myself when I remember how I used to make fun of the 'hotflash club.' Live and learn I guess. Now if these estrogen shots would just give me back my sex drive, things wouldn't be so bad. The doctor tells me there's no reason for it but his nurse told me privately that lots of women complain about the same thing.

Hormones work. They not only make a woman feel better herself, they improve her perception of other people. Esther A., an independent CPA, put it even more succinctly: "When I need my shot, look out, world!"

While hormones do many wonderful things, sexual dysfunction—which includes lack of desire—will not be changed by hormone therapy. Lorraine Dennerstein, senior lecturer in the Department of Psychiatry of the University of Melbourne and president of the Australian Society for Psychosomatic Obstetrics and Gynecology, advises that proper sexual counseling is needed and, if the woman is married or has a regular partner, the couple should be seen together.

Sixty percent of the male partners of sexually distressed women also suffer sexual dysfunction, she says, with many of the male partner's problems stemming from his belief that his wife is rejecting him because she is no longer being aroused. He reacts with anger, which tends to diminish his erectile capabilities. When the couple does attempt intercourse, they're uncomfortable with one another, they're both in a hurry to get it over with so they tend to cut down on foreplay, which makes matters worse. The man's major concern is the woman's lack of sexual arousal—so different than before her surgery. A woman who has lost her ovaries requires far more direct stimulation to become aroused. This should be a very pleasurable part of lovemaking; things can slow down and this need not be a disadvantage as long as the couple understands what is happening.

Physical fitness is closely tied to self-image, which can be extremely important in sexual response. A woman who keeps herself well-groomed is likely to have a better self-image than the woman who ignores her appearance. Recent studies show that women who look younger than their age, are physically fit, and feel youthful actually do live longer and enjoy better health. While activity and medical fitness have not been examined specifically in relation to sexuality, perhaps they will be in the future.

Hypnosis has proven amazingly helpful in treating sexual dysfunction brought about by surgery. There are now a few gynecological surgeons who employ brief clinical hypnosis techniques with excellent results.

Dr. David B. Cheek, who conducts a busy gynecological practice in San Francisco, says that much is gained by the surgeon who takes the time to prepare a woman mentally and emotionally in advance of her operation, adding that the job is made easier for the surgeon who knows that radical surgery need not necessarily end the sexual life of a patient, even when vulva and clitoris and vagina have been removed. He adds that re-education is more difficult when it has to be started during the postoperative period against the handicap of deeply imprinted convictions that have occurred while the patient is unconscious with a general anesthetic.

One of Dr. Cheek's patients, a young woman in her late twenties, suffered from cancer of the vulva, which is very rare in women of this age. The cancer was so advanced by the time she went to Dr. Cheek that it was necessary for him to perform a radical vulvectomy including removal of her rectum, lower vagina, vulva, clitoris and lower mons veneris. Understandably, the young woman was stunned by the knowledge that she had a life-threatening cancer, and did not seem to grasp the enormity of the surgery that would be involved—a spontaneously occurring denial mechanism that often protects such patients from suicidal thoughts at time of crisis.

For two days prior to the surgery, Dr. Cheek worked with the sexual attitudes of the patient while using hypnosis to prepare her for surgery and the recovery period. He learned that she had been sexually responsive before the onset of her disease, capable of multiple orgasms during intercourse. He told her that her earlier happy sexual experiences had set images in her mind that were permanent and would be available to her in the future. To demonstrate to her how much her mind could alter awareness and at the same time alter reaction to tissue injury, he placed her in a light hypnotic state and asked her to remember how one arm would feel if she had been lying on it and it had gone to sleep. After she was aware that there really was a difference in feeling between her arms, he made a scratch on each arm from the wrist upward.

Then he spent about fifteen minutes telling her the various steps in the surgery and what she would be expected to do afterwards in order to gain mobility, feel hungry and eliminate easily from her bladder and bowel.

When this was over, the young patient was pleased and surprised to discover that the scratch made on the "numb" arm was almost invisible while the scratch on the other arm was red and puffy. Dr. Cheek explained that if there is pain in a wound, the healing process is delayed because fresh blood cannot get near to remove waste products and add oxygen and nutrition necessary for the process of repair and the antibiotics in her blood wouldn't have a chance to work where they were most needed.

This seemed reasonable to the patient. She was hypnotized again and quickly responded to the suggestion that she had walked into cold water and had been standing there long enough to feel numb as well as cold. She nodded acceptance to the suggestion that she could do this any time she wanted and that she understood the deeper tissues would also feel cool and numb on command and could remain that way for at least two hours. After being told about the value of eating properly after surgery, she practiced remembering a time when she had felt very hungry, soon her stomach was growling and she remembered the pleasant feeling of fullness after a delicious imagined meal.

Then Dr. Cheek moved into a convincing exercise with sexual memories. She had often had sexual dreams ending in orgasm. He pointed out that there is no genital contact during such dreams, that she must practice not only dreaming in her sleep but also remembering in hypnosis all the pleasurable feelings she had known during intercourse. This must be done, he said, to speed up the return of sensation to her pelvic area during her recovery period. She was asked to select a particularly good memory from the past and let Dr. Cheek know by nodding her head when she felt a "subconscious" climax. He reports that not only did she nod, but it was clear from her respiration and unconscious hip motions that she had an excellent memory.

Just before going into the operating room, she was again placed into a hypnotic state and asked to make her body and legs cool and numb, and to think about this coolness immediately on awakening after surgery. The operation took four hours. The packing was removed from the space left by the rectum and vagina on the second postoperative day.

At a follow-up visit to the doctor's office it was clear that the patient had accepted her colostomy and was glad to be alive. Dr. Cheek placed her in hypnosis again and rehearsed her with memories of a particularly pleasurable sexual experience, asking her to relive this several times while he was out of the room examining other patients. He stressed that a most important part of her recovery involved the frequent use of self-hypnosis and the reliving of sexually satisfying experiences—that doing so would help sensation return to her genital area and would be helpful in keeping the scar tissue soft and pliable.

Dr. Cheek reports that nine years later this woman walked into his office looking young, pretty, and happy. She was now married. She told him that she had multiple orgasms during foreplay, that she had more feeling in her dimple of a vagina than she had ever had before with all her equipment intact.

"The discussions about sexual responsiveness were initially considered only a part of a larger-scale drive to keep this young woman from dwelling on the enormity of her immediate problem by giving her confidence that she could survive the ordeal and aim for future goals of normal function as a female," Dr. Cheek says. "Apparently some shreds of ovarian tissue must have remained after removal of her tubo-ovarian inflammatory masses, for she had no vasomotor disturbances to suggest that she had entered a premature menopause."

In another case involving hypnosis, a twenty-two-year-old nurse went for a routine annual checkup with her gynecologist. She had just established her independence financially, was happy in her work, was dating and looking forward to marriage.

During the examination, her gynecologist found a suspicious lesion in the vagina anterior to the cervix. He asked if her mother had ever taken diethylstilbestrol. She had. Biopsy of the vaginal lesion substantiated the gynecologist's fears. He called her with the shocking news that she would have to have a hysterectomy and complete removal of the vagina combined with a radical gland dissection, adding that because of the position of the lesion it might also be necessary to remove the bladder and make an artificial bladder with a segment of small bowel. If this were the case, her bladder would then open through her abdomen into a bag.

She went into an emotional blackout. It seemed to her that this must be happening to someone else. She could take no action, make no decisions for several days. Her preparation for heroic surgery consisted of a dazzlingly clear outline of the possible complications. She would have to accept the fact that she would have no children. There could be no guarantee that she would remain cancer-free after surgery. Her physician could not promise to save her bladder; he would have to see if the bladder had been invaded by the vaginal cancer. Her questions about what would happen to her sex life were fielded deftly but not answered.

Her uterus, vagina, and one ovary were removed. After surgery, she developed a urinary tract infection. The constant saturation of her bed with urine was first ascribed to leakage around the Foley catheter until it was discovered that she had direct drainage from a defect in the bladder wall communicating with the space once occupied by her vagina. In addition to the bladder drainage, she had no control over her anal sphincter. Instead of offering positive advice about what could be done to correct these problems, her surgeon became unpleasantly defensive. She went home wearing rubber pants, a useless catheter in her bladder and multiple heavy-duty sanitary pads to mop up excess urine. Later, she fell into an even deeper depression with the discovery that she could not reach a climax with masturbation. Her clitoris was anesthetic.

When she asked her surgeon about this, his answer was that it was *her* problem because he had not cut any nerves to her clitoris. He continued to assert that the bladder openings would close in time. Months passed. During the following year she consulted seven urologists, all to no avail.

At this point she reluctantly accepted her father's request that she consult Dr. Cheek in the hope that hypnosis might relieve some of the discomfort of surgery and perhaps aid in the healing process. She was skeptical about the value of hypnosis and had never accepted her father's interest in it. Her need was so great, however, that she went to see Dr. Cheek. Fortunately there had been two other doctors who had told her that damaged pelvic nerves can sometimes grow back. Under hypnosis, she accepted Dr. Cheek's statement that their job was to hook up the circuits of feeling again and that the process would be greatly accelerated if she learned to use self-hypnosis and would practice remembering pleasurable sensations as they had been in the past.

Then she was asked to rehearse some familiar experiences not specifically related to her immediate problems; she was asked to remember hunger followed by a feeling of fullness, thirst followed by a satisfying drink. Eventually she was told to go back in time to some period of her life when she had experienced a sex dream ending in orgasm. With just brief practice, she was able to experience orgasm in dreams and with masturbation.

During the following year she underwent several operations that successfully closed the bladder fistulae and gave her control over her sphincter. She married the thoughtful and understanding man who had stood by her during this terrible time. Her sex life is normal and rewarding and she is now working with disabled and discouraged people.

179

A New Kind of Doctor

Women ask if it would be better to have only female doctors. Would they have more understanding in dealing with hysterectomy?

Not necessarily. Understanding and awareness depend on more than the sex of the doctor. Both male and female doctors must rise above their traditional training that equates perfection with cutting and amputation. Both female and male doctors are products of medical schools, of traditional medical thinking; both are heirs to the dead hand rule.

In the 1950s well over 90 percent of the physicians in the United States were men. Now, in most medical schools, one-third of the students are women. As far as academic medicine is concerned, and given the tenure system, women have a long way to go. Their advance will be slow. At the present time, department chairmen at medical schools across the country are all men. Women, estimated to make up between 5 and 10 percent of medical faculties nationwide, are clustered at the bottom of the ladder.

Women gynecologists, however, are moving speedily into private practice and are attracting new patients faster than men do. Estimates are that by 1990 one out of five practicing gynecologists will be a woman.

Whether man or woman, what is desperately needed are Woman-Doctors, both male and female, who understand women's specialness, who know how to treat a woman as a woman. Because women are female, they are different. It is their hormonal makeup that causes this to be so. They have their own health problems that are not always centered in the gynecological area. For example, because of women's special chemistry, female alcoholics become addicted more quickly than do male alcoholics. Women suffer more damage from alcoholism and take longer to recover. They are more prone to back problems. Caffeine is more harmful to them. Even medications used by men and women for the same ailments may cause far more severe reactions in women.

What women need are Woman-Doctors who understand and practice holistic medicine (the *whole* body), who will help women save the organs that make them women, who will understand sexual enrichment as a motivating force in their lives. Women need Woman-Doctors who are caring enough so that they can feel comfortable discussing sensitive issues. Above all, women need Woman-Doctors who will tell them the truth. One of women's major human rights is the right to be completely and truthfully informed about their bodies.

There *are* enlightened physicians about the country, doctors who are in tune with real women, physicians who are Woman-Doctors. Outstanding among these is Dr. Peter Bours who practices in his own clinic in Forest Grove, a small town located in western Oregon.

Dr. Bours is a tall bearded man in his early forties. An economics major at Stanford University, Peter Bours did his senior thesis on population control and economic development in third-world countries. It was an interest he brought from home—his parents had long been active in Planned Parenthood—and it decided him on a career in medicine. After graduation from Harvard Medical School, he signed on as an intern at the University of California in San Diego. He had planned to become an orthopedic surgeon, but during his internship and residence in San Diego he became fascinated with the care of children and families. He decided that when he began to practice, it would be in family and woman care.

His search for a redefinition of personal and social relationships led him to Forest Grove, where he was drawn by the uncomplicated grandeur of the country. In 1974 he bought a piece of farmland and an old frame house outside the town and went into practice. Within a few years he married his nurse, Joan Moss, and together they built a family practice at first based on delivering babies, often to couples who wanted their children born at home or in one of the birthing cabins that Dr. Bours built on his property. Few doctors were offering that kind of care, and before long Joan and Peter Bours had hundreds of couples from Portland traveling the thirty miles to have their babies. Keeping his rates low, paying himself a comparatively small salary, he sank the rest of his income into a clinic across the street from the community hospital. The clinic is remarkable for its friendly, informal atmosphere. Part of the clinic has been devoted to birthing; a large comfortable sitting room, convenient kitchen, and several good-sized rooms with adjustable beds comprise the area where babies are delivered in a home-like atmosphere. The family can be present. The woman labors and delivers in the same bed with the support of those she loves at her side. There is no feeling that birthing is an illness; rather it is welcomed as a joyous natural event. To the despair of many, Dr. Bours is giving up delivering babies, after well over two thousand births. In Oregon, insurance premiums for doctors doing birthing have risen from $6,000 to $30,000 a year and will keep rising. But without the birthing, all of his energies will be focused on woman care, from age five on.

Peter Bours is a different sort of doctor. He presents himself casually, and all of his patients call him by his first name. "I can talk about anything with Peter," said one young woman whose four children had been delivered by Dr. Bours. "He understands what makes a woman tick."

What does this woman's health-care specialist think about hysterectomy? He doesn't like it. "In all my years of practice I've only done two hysterectomies and they were that rarity, matters of life or death," he said. "I don't believe in hysterectomy. It can tear up a woman's whole life. I believe in treating the condition. It's about time we start applying fair standards. If we're going to do hysterectomies for some of the reasons doctors do them, then we'd better start taking out men's prostates for their aches and pains."

Dr. Peter Bours, when asked how a woman can personally combat the epidemic of hysterectomy sweeping the country, replied: "First of all, a woman must arm herself with a few basic facts about hysterectomy, like when it is absolutely necessary and when it is not. Then she must look for a gynecologist whose first response is not surgery. If she has a good relationship with her family physician and he or she is someone the woman can trust and one who knows her family, she should consider using her family physician as an advocate between her and the gynecologist. In this way, the family physician can make the gynecologist justify his reasons for hysterectomy."

Peter Bours is a good physician. The *other* good physician is a woman herself. Women have a duty to themselves to learn as much as possible about their own bodies and to be certain that their daughters learn about *their* own bodies. As a society, Americans tend to be superficial, wanting to know how to do everything from achieving expert orgasm to running a computer in ten easy steps. But today's busy woman—*especially* today's woman—must take the time and energy to learn about her own body. Human sexuality courses are offered through many universities and community colleges. Women's health centers teach classes in self-examination during which women are taught how to use the various gynecological instruments, how to examine themselves, and how to recognize what they are looking for.

Women must take responsibility for knowing enough about their bodies so that they won't be sold an operation they don't need. Even if removal of the uterus is necessary, concurrent removal of the ovaries is usually unnecessary and certainly undesirable, and should be expressly forbidden by the patient when she signs the operation permit.

Some say that hysterectomy is only surgical menopause and that every woman has to go through menopause. (The word *menopause* is frequently misused; it actually means the last period.) Nothing could be further from the truth. Castration precipitates a woman into immediate physical problems that are not shared by women who undergo a natural menopause with healthy bodies, unimpaired metabolism, intact endocrine systems, and undamaged genitalia. Natural menopause is one of many transitional phases of normal female life; the normal menopausal woman has not suffered "ovarian death" or "outlived her ovaries," two common and inaccurate descriptions. There is, to the contrary, evidence of ovarian function during the years after menopause and well into old age and, while not adequate to sustain fertility, certainly present in large enough quantities to permit a woman to still be who and what she was premenopausally, possessing her own unique physical and mental characteristics.

Contrary to the popular myth of the menopausal woman, a recent study of more than eight thousand menopausal women conducted by The American Institutes for Research in the Behavioral Sciences of Cambridge, Massachusetts, indicates that the stereotype of the depressed, unstable, hypochondriacal menopausal woman is just *not so*. Women who haven't been "cut" usually get along fine.

Of the eight thousand women studied, the 30 percent who had undergone hysterectomy reported more chronic illness, used twice as many prescribed drugs, had more surgery for benign breast disease and, in general, felt in poorer health, sought professional help more often, and had less education than the 70 percent who experienced natural menopause. The conclusion reached by epidemiologist Sonja M. McKinlay: That menopause neither increases illness nor fosters any undue use of medical care, *except* when it is caused by the scalpel rather than by the biological clock.

When women become knowledgeable about their own bodies, and when enlightened, concerned Woman-Doctors are available for counsel and support, hysterectomy will be a surgery of the past.

Epilogue

After talking with many women who had also suffered disquieting and sometimes terrifying aftereffects of hysterectomy, I began to feel better about myself.

I realized that I was not the only woman who suffered in these ways; that it was, in fact, an actual medical condition—post-hysterectomy syndrome. Contrary to what many doctors had told me, I was not alone. I was not crazy, not "overly-imaginative," nor even necessarily "over-sexed," as one doctor solemnly told me. I was a woman who had been castrated.

This knowledge made me draw closer to my husband. Always a tower of strength in my life, he now became my best friend, the one person I could talk to without inhibition. Eventually, we both had to accept the fact that if we hadn't allowed ourselves to become panic-stricken at Dr. Jones's words of doom—if we had waited for Dr. Hara—I would not have undergone the surgery. We accepted this and then let go of any guilt, of any "if onlies."

We determined to rebuild our emotional lives. Joe was reassured that I hadn't lost interest in him and I was reassured that some irresistible woman with all her parts wouldn't seize his attention. We knew we had each other, probably in a deeper sense than ever before. He not only encouraged me to write a book about the aftereffects of hysterectomy, he actually helped me with my research, talking to a number of men whose wives had undergone the same experience. As our emotional life mended and became stronger, so did our intimate life become different and even more rewarding. Everything each of us did was for the other.

Not long ago, a doctor I was interviewing asked me what *The Castrated Woman* was about. I was silent for a while, thinking: It's about my experience and other women's experiences with the surgery, it's about facts and figures, and medical research. Suddenly I realized what the book is really about.

"It's about love," I replied.

"Love?" he asked, puzzled.

"Love," I said. "Love of a woman for her own body, enough to prevent it from being thoughtlessly mutilated. And the love of her partner, enough love to surmount the difficulties hysterectomy presents."

For Further Information

Those interested in hypnotherapy treatment for sexual dysfunction may write to the following organization for recommended members in their area:

American Society of Clinical Hypnosis
2250 Devon Avenue, Suite 336
Des Plaines, IL 60018

Current information regarding all phases of hysterectomy may be obtained by writing to:

Nora Coffey
HERS
Hysterectomy Educational Resources and Services
422 Brynmawr Avenue
Balacynwyd, PA 19004

Caution should be used when choosing a sex therapist. Since many states do not require licensing of marriage counselors and sex therapists, potential clients should protect themselves by investigating the counselor's qualifications. Try to find a therapist who is a member of an organization which requires a masters degree or doctorate and supervised training; certification by the American Association of Sex Educators, Counselors and Therapists; or licensing by the state's pyschiatric, psychological, or social worker boards.

Also, beware of someone who has just moved into the community; a therapist who touches you, invites disrobing or suggests home visits; being forced to engage in activities against your own philosophy or religious beliefs; anyone who makes you feel uneasy; questionable hypnotic practices, such as being massaged while under hypnosis; long-term therapy. Most sexual therapy is of short duration.

Those wishing more information regarding endometriosis are invited to write to:

Endometriosis Association
PO Box 92187
Milwaukee, WI 53202

Bibliography

Books

Abelow, Dan. *Total Sex.* New York: Grossett and Dunlap, 1976.

Airola, Paavo. *Every Woman's Book.* Phoenix, AZ: Health Plus, 1979.

Barbach, Lonnie and Linda Levine. *Shared Intimacies.* New York: Anchor Press, 1980.

Bardwick, J. M. *Psychology of Women.* New York: Harper and Row, 1971.

Beach, Frank A. *Human Sexuality in Four Perspectives.* Baltimore: The Johns Hopkins University Press, 1976.

Beauvoir, Simone de. *The Second Sex.* New York: Alfred A. Knopf, 1952.

Belliveau, Fred and Lin Richter. *Understanding Human Sexual Inadequacy.* Boston: Little, Brown, 1970.

Bermant, Gordon and Julian M. Davidson. *Biological Bases of Sexual Behavior.* New York: Harper and Row, 1974.

Bettelheim, Bruno. *The Uses of Enchantment: The Meaning and Importance of Fairy Tales.* New York: Thames and Hudson, 1976.

———. *Symbolic Wounds: Puberty Rites and the Envious Male.* New York: Thames and Hudson, 1955.

Blumstein, Philip and Pepper Schwartz. *American Couples.* New York: William Morrow, 1983.

Bodanis, David. *The Body Book.* Boston: Little, Brown, 1984.

Boston Women's Health Book Collective. *Our Bodies, Ourselves.* New York: Simon and Schuster, 1971.

Boston Women's Health Book Collective. *The New Our Bodies, Ourselves.* New York: Simon and Schuster, 1984.

Brecher, Edward M. and the editors of Consumer Reports Books. *Love, Sex and Aging.* Boston: Little, Brown, 1984.

Brecher, Edward M. *The Sex Researchers.* San Francisco: Specific Press, 1969.

Brody, Jane. *The New York Times Guide to Personal Health*. New York: Times Books, 1976.

Brownmiller, Susan. *Against Our Will: Men, Women and Rape*. New York: Simon and Schuster, 1975.

Campbell, B. *Sexual Selection and the Descent of Man*. Hawthorne, NY: Aldine, 1972.

Carrera, Michael. *Sex: The Facts, the Acts and Your Feelings*. New York: Crown, 1981.

Cassell, Carol. *Swept Away: Why Women Fear Their Own Sexuality*. New York: Simon and Schuster, 1984.

Chamberlain, Mary. *Old Wives' Tales*. London: Virago Press, 1981.

Comfort, Alex. *The Joy of Sex*. New York: Simon and Schuster, 1972.

Cooke, Cynthia and Susan Dworkin. *The MS. Guide to Women's Health*. New York: Anchor Books, 1979.

Cooper, Wendy. *Don't Change*. New York: Stein and Day, 1975.

Corea, Gena. *The Hidden Malpractice: How American Medicine Mistreats Women*. New York: Berkley Publishing Groups, 1977.

Cutler, Winifred Berg, Celso-Ramon Garcia, and David A. Edwards. *Menopause*. New York: Norton, 1983.

Daly, Mary. *Pure Lust*. Boston: Beacon Press, 1984.

Davidson, J. M. *Hormones and Behavior*. New York: Academic Press, 1972.

Davies, Nigel. *The Rampant God*. New York: William Morrow, 1984.

Deaton, John G., Elizabeth Jean Pascoe, and Philip R. Alper. *The Woman's Day Book of Family Medical Questions*. New York: Random House, 1979.

Demetrakopoulos, Stephanie. *Listening to Our Bodies: The Rebirth of Feminine Wisdom*. Boston: Beacon Press, 1983.

Driver, Harold E. *Indians of North America*. Chicago: University of Chicago Press, 1960.

Edelstein, L. *Greek Medicine*. Baltimore: The Johns Hopkins University Press, 1967.

Ehrenreich, Barbara and Deirdre English. *For Her Own Good*. New York: Anchor Press, 1978.

Gawthorne-Hardy, Jonathan. *Marriage, Love, Sex and Divorce*. New York: Summit Books, 1981.

Gifford-Jones, W. *On Being a Woman*. New York: Macmillan, 1969.

———. *What Every Woman Should Know About Hysterectomy*. New York: Funk and Wagnalls, 1977.

Giustini, F. G., and S. J. Keefer. *Understanding Hysterectomy: A Woman's Guide*. New York: Walker, 1979.

Gold, Jay J. *Gynaecologic Endocrinology*. New York: Harper and Row, 1975.

Gould, George M. and Walter L. Pyle. *Anomalies and Curiosities of Medicine*. New York: Crown, 1975.

Greer, Germaine. *The Female Eunuch*. New York: McGraw-Hill, 1970.

Hamilton, Eleanor. *Partners in Love*. San Diego: A. S. Barnes, 1961.

Harrison, Michelle. *A Woman in Residence*. New York: Random House, 1982.

Heath, Stephen. *The Sexual Fix*. New York: Schocken, 1984.

Hesler, Phyllis C. *Women and Madness*. New York: Doubleday, 1972.

Hogbin, Ian. *The Island of Menstruating Men: Religion in Wogeo, New Guinea*. London: Chandler, Scranton, 1970.

Holt, Linda Hughey and Melva Weber. *The American Medical Association book of WOMAN CARE*. New York: Random House, 1981.

Huneycutt, Harry C. and Judith L. David. *All About Hysterectomy*. New York: The Dial Press, 1977.

Jaffe, Dennis T. *Healing from Within*. New York: Alfred A. Knopf, 1980.

Jayne, Walter. *The Healing Gods of Ancient Civilizations*. New Haven, CT: Yale University Press, 1915.

Joy, Brugh W. *Joy's Way: An Introduction to the Potentials for Healing with Body Energies*. Los Angeles: J. P. Tarcher, 1979.

Kaufman, Sherwin A. *From a Gynecologist's Notebook*. New York: Stein and Day, 1974.

Kinsey, A. C., W. Pomeroy, C. Martin and P. Gebhard. *Sexual Behavior in the Human Female*. Philadelphia: Saunders, 1953.

Kitzinger, Sheila. *Woman's Experience of Sex*. New York: Putnam's, 1983.

Kramer, Ann. *A Woman's Body: An Owner's Manual*. New York: Grossett and Dunlap, 1977.

Ladas, Alice Kahn, Beverly Whipple and John D. Perry. *The G Spot*. New York: Dell, 1981.

Lair, Jess. *Sex: If I Didn't Laugh I'd Cry*. New York: Doubleday, 1979.

Lake, Alice. *Our Own Years: What Women Over 35 Should Know About Themselves*. Minneapolis: Winston Press, 1979.

Lerner, Gerda. *The Female Experience*. Indianapolis: Bobbs-Merrill, 1977.

Levine, R. L. *Endocrines and the Central Nervous System*. Baltimore: Williams and Wilkins, 1966.

Liebowitz, Michael R. *The Chemistry of Love*. Boston: Little, Brown, 1983.

Llewellyn-Jones, Derek. *Everywoman and Her Body*. New York: Taplinger, 1971.

Lowen, Alexander. *Depression and the Body*. New York: Coward McCann and Geoghegan, 1972.

Maccoby, E. E., and C. M. Jacklin. *The Psychology of Sex Differences*. San Francisco: Stanford University Press, 1974.

Madaras, Lynda, and Jane Patterson. *Womancare*. New York: Avon, 1981.

Marshall, D. S., and R. C. Suggs. *Human Sexual Behavior: Variations in the Ethnographic Spectrum*. Englewood Cliffs, NJ: Prentice-Hall, 1972.

Martini, L., and W. F. Ganong. *Frontiers in Neuroendocrinology*. New York: Oxford University Press, 1971.

Masters, William H. and Virginia E. Johnson, *Human Sexual Inadequacy*. Boston: Little, Brown, 1970.

———. *Human Sexual Response*. Boston: Little, Brown, 1966.

191

Masters, William H. and Virginia E. Johnson. *The Pleasure Bond.* Boston: Little, Brown, 1975.

Mattingly, R. F., ed. *TeLinde's Operative Gynecology,* 5th ed. Philadelphia: Lippincott, 1977.

McKay, W. J. Stewart. *A History of Ancient Gynaecology.* London: Bailliere, Tindall-Cox, 1901.

Mead, Margaret. *Male and Female.* New York: William Morrow, 1949.

Mendelsohn, Robert S. *Confessions of a Medical Heretic.* Chicago: Contemporary Books, 1979.

―――. *MALePRACTICE: How Doctors Manipulate Women.* Chicago: Contemporary Books, 1981.

Michael, R., ed. *Endocrinology and Human Behavior.* New York: Oxford University Press, 1968.

Miller, Jonathan. *The Body in Question.* New York: Random House, 1978.

Montagna, W., and W. A. Sadler. *Reproductive Behavior.* New York: Plenum Press, 1974.

Montagu, Ashley. *Touching.* New York: Harper and Row, 1972.

Morgan, Elaine. *The Descent of Woman.* New York: Stein and Day, 1972.

Morgan, Susanne. *Coping with a Hysterectomy.* New York: Dial, 1982.

Offit, Avodah K. *The Sexual Self.* New York: Lippincott, 1977.

Penney, Alexandra. *How to Make Love to a Man.* New York: Clarkson N. Potter, 1981.

Phillips, Debora and Robert Judd. *Sexual Confidence.* Boston: Houghton Mifflin, 1980.

Pietropinto, Anthony and Jacqueline Simenauer. *Husbands and Wives.* New York: Times Books, 1979.

Prevention Magazine editors. *Surgery and Its Alternatives.* Emmaus, PA: Rodale Press, 1980.

Progoff, Ira. *At a Journal Workshop.* New York: Dialogue House Library, 1975.

Rivers, W. H. R. *Medicine, Magic and Religion.* London: (self-published), 1924.

Sagan, Carl. *Broca's Brain.* New York: Random House, 1974.

Sarrel, Lorna G., and Phillip M. Sarrel. *Sexual Turning Points.* New York: Macmillan, 1984.

Savramis, Demosthenes. *The Satanizing of Woman: Religion Versus Sexuality.* New York: Doubleday, 1974.

Scheimann, Eugene. *Sex Can Save Your Heart and Life.* New York: Crown, 1974.

Seaman, Barbara and Gideon Seaman. *Women and the Crisis in Sex Hormones.* New York: Rawson Associates, 1977.

Shainess, Natalie. *Sweet Suffering.* New York: Bobbs-Merrill, 1983.

Shephard, Bruce D. and Carroll A. Shephard. *The Complete Guide to Women's Health.* New York: Mariner, 1982.

Shuttle, Penelope and Peter Redgrove. *The Wise Wound.* New York: Richard Marek, 1978.

Silverman, Hirsch Lazaar. *Marital Therapy.* New York: Charles C. Thomas, 1972.

Sisley, Emily L. and Bertha Harris. *The Joy of Lesbian Sex.* New York: Crown, 1977.

Sommers, Sheldon C. *Genital and Mammary Pathology Decennial.* New York: Appleton-Century-Crofts, 1975.

Stewart, Felicia. *My Body, My Health.* New York: John Wiley, 1979.

Stoppard, Miriam. *Being a Well Woman.* New York: Holt, Rinehart and Winston, 1982.

Sweeney, William J., III, with Barbara Lang Stern. *Woman's Doctor.* New York: William Morrow, 1973.

Symons, Donald. *The Evolution of Human Sexuality.* New York: Oxford University Press, 1979.

Tannahill, Reay. *Sex in History.* New York: Stein and Day, 1980.

Tart, Charles T. *Altered States of Consciousness.* New York: Anchor Books, 1972.

Washburn, S. L. and R. Moore. *Ape into Man: A Study of Human Evolution.* Boston: Little, Brown, 1974.

Weideger, Paula. *Menstruation and Menopause.* New York: Alfred A. Knopf, 1975.

Whalen, R. E. *Hormones and Behavior.* New York: Van Nostrand, 1967.

Wilson, Robert A. *Feminine Forever.* New York: M. Evans, 1966.

Witkin-Lanoil, Georgia. *The Female Stress System.* New York: Newmarket Press, 1984.

Wolf, Linda. *The Cosmo Report.* New York: Arbor House, 1981.

Young, W. C., ed. *Sex and Internal Secretions.* New York: Williams and Wilkins, 1961.

Articles

Ahdieh, Harry B. and George N. Wade. 1982. "Effects of hysterectomy on sexual receptivity, food intake, running wheel activity, and hypothalamic estrogen and progestin receptors in rats." *Journal of Comparative and Physiological Psychology.* Vol. 96: 886–892.

Atkinson, S. M. and S. M. Chappell. 1972. "Vaginal hysterectomy for sterilization." *Obstetrics and Gynecology.* Vol. 39: 759–766.

Auchincloss, S. S. 1971. "Dream content and the menstrual cycle." Honors thesis, Harvard University.

Bassin, Donna. 1982. "Woman's images of inner space: data towards expanded interpretive categories." *International Review of Psychoanalysis.* Vol. 9: 191–203.

Beach, F. A. 1975. "Behavioral endocrinology: An emerging discipline." *American Scientist.* Vol. 63: 178–187.

———. 1976. "Sexual attractivity, proceptivity and receptivity in female mammals." *Hormonal Behavior.* Vol. 7: 105–138.

Berry, Constance and Frederick L. McGuire. 1972. "Menstrual distress and acceptance of sexual role." *American Journal of Obstetrics and Gynecology.* Vol. 114: 83–87.

Biondi, C. and S. Zolesi. 1980. "Considerations of the psychological attitude of patients awaiting hysterectomy." *Psichiatria Generale e dell'Eta Evolutiva.* Vol. 18: 411–417.

Brown, Frank A. 1972. "The 'clocks' timing biological rhythms." *American Scientist.* (November-December): 756–766.

Brown, Judith. 1963. "A cross-cultural study of female initiation rites." *American Anthropologist.* Vol. 65: 837–853.

Brush, Louise A. 1938. "Attitudes, emotional and physical symptoms commonly associated with menstruation in 100 women." *The American Journal of Orthopsychiatry.* Vol. 8: 286–301.

Burr, H. S. and L. K. Musselman. 1936. "Bio-electric phenomena associated with menstruation." *Yale Journal of Biology and Medicine.* Vol. 9: 155–158.

Centerwall, B. S. 1981. "Premenopausal hysterectomy and cardiovascular disease." *American Journal of Obstetrics and Gynecology.* Vol. 139: 58–61.

Cheek, David B. 1976. "Hypnotherapy for secondary frigidity after radical surgery for gynecological cancer: Two case reports." *American Journal of Clinical Hypnosis.* (July): 13–19.

Chevalier-Skolnikoff, S. 1974. "Male-female, female-female, male-male sexual behavior in the stumptail monkey, with special attention to the female orgasm." *Archives of Sexual Behavior.* Vol. 3: 95–116.

Coleman, Emily M., Peter W. Hoon and Emily F. Hoon. 1983. "Arousability and sexual satisfaction in lesbian and heterosexual women." *Journal of Sex Research.* Vol. 19: 58–73.

Comarr, A. E. 1970. "Sexual function among patients with spinal cord injury." *Urologia Internationalis.* Vol. 25: 134.

"A Comparison of Operations and Surgeons in the United States and in England and Wales." 1970. *New England Journal of Medicine.* Vol. 282: 135.

Copenhaver, E. H. 1962. "Vaginal hysterectomy: An analysis of indications and complications among 1,000 operations." *American Journal of Obstetrics and Gynecology.* Vol. 84: 123–128.

Coppen, A. and N. Kessel. 1963. "Menstruation and personality." *British Journal of Psychiatry.* Vol. 109: 711–721.

Cyck, F., F. A. Murphy, J. K. Murphy, et al. 1977. "Effect of surveillance on the number of hysterectomies in the Province of Saskatchewan." *New England Journal of Medicine*. Vol. 296: 1326–1328.

Davidson, Julian M. 1981. "The Orgasmic Connection." *Psychology Today*. (July): 91.

deBarenne, Dorothea D. and Frederick A. Gibbs. 1942. "Variations in the electroencephalogram during the menstrual cycle." *American Journal of Obstetrics and Gynecology*. Vol. 4: 687–690.

deBruijn, Gerda. 1982. "From masturbation to orgasm with a partner: How some women bridge the gap—and why others don't." *Journal of Sex and Marital Therapy*. Vol. 8: 151–167.

Degen, Kathleen. 1982. "Sexual dysfunction in women using major tranquilizers." *Psychosomatics*. Vol. 23: 959–961.

Dennerstein, L. and C. Wood, et al. 1977. "Sexual response following hysterectomy and oophorectomy." *Obstetrics and Gynecology*. Vol. 49: 92–96.

Diamond, M. 1965. "A critical evaluation of the ontogeny of human sexual behavior." *Quarterly Review of Biology*. Vol. 40: 147–75.

Diamond, Milton, Leonard A. Diamond and Marian Mast. 1972. "Visual sensitivity and sexual arousal levels during the menstrual cycle." *The Journal of Nervous and Mental Disease*. Vol. 155: 170–176.

Dicker, Richard C., Mark J. Scalley, Joel R. Greenspan, Peter M. Layde, Howard W. Ory, Joyce M. Maze and Jack C. Smith. 1982. "Hysterectomy among women of reproductive age." *Journal of the American Medical Association*. Vol. 248 (July): 323–327.

Doyle, J. C. 1953. "Unnecessary hysterectomies: Study of 6,248 operations in 35 hospitals during 1948." *Journal of the American Medical Association*. Vol. 151: 360–365.

Easterday, Charles L., David A. Grimes and Joseph A. Riggs. 1983. "Hysterectomy in the United States." *Obstetrics and Gynecology*. Vol. 62 (August): 203–212.

Everett, B. J. and J. Herbert. 1969. "Adrenal glands and sexual receptivity of female rhesus monkeys." *Journal of Endocrincology*. Vol. 51: 575–588.

———. 1970. "The maintenance of sexual receptivity by adrenal androgens in female rhesus monkeys." *Journal of Endocrinology*. Vol. 48: 892–895.

Fisher, Charles. 1983. "Patterns of female sexual arousal during sleep and waking: Vaginal thermo-conductance studies." *Archives of Sexual Behavior*. Vol. 12: 97–122.

Frenkel, Richard E. 1971. "Remembering dreams through autosuggestion relationship of menstruation and ovulation to the autosuggestion dream recall cycle." *Behavioural Neuropsychiatry*. Vol. 3: 2–11.

Gath, Dennis, Peter Cooper and Ann Day. 1982. "Hysterectomy and psychiatric disorder: 1. levels of psychiatric morbidity before and after hysterectomy." *British Journal of Psychiatry*. Vol. 140: 335–342.

Goldberg, Daniel C., et al. 1983. "The Grafenberg Spot and female ejaculation: a review of initial hypothesis." *Journal of Sex and Marital Therapy*. Vol. 9: 27–37.

Harris, G. W., and R. P. Michael. 1964. "The activation of sexual behavior by hypothalamic implants of estrogen." *Journal of Physiology*. Vol. 171: 275.

Hart, R. D. 1960. "Monthly rhythm of libido in married women." *British Medical Journal*. Vol. 1: 1023–1024.

Henson, Donald E., H. B. Rubin, and Claudia Henson. 1982. "Labial and vaginal blood volume response to visual and tactile stimuli." *Archives of Sexual Behavior*. Vol. 11: 23–31.

Hoon, Peter W., Emily Coleman, Janis Amberson and Frank Ling. 1981. "A possible physiological marker of female sexual dysfunction." *Biological Psychiatry*. Vol. 16: 1101–1106.

Hori, T., M. Ide and T. Miyake. 1968. "Ovarian estrogen secretion during the estrous cycle and under the influence of exogenous gonadotropins in rats." *Endocrinology in Japan*. Vol. 15: 215.

"International Panel Discussion: Role of Hormone Therapy in Osteoporosis and Sexual Dysfunction." 1983. *The Female Patient*. Vol. 8 (August): 32/1–32/10.

Johnson, G. B. 1932. "The effects of periodicity on learning to walk a tightwire." *Comparative Psychology*. Vol. 13: 133–141.

Jost, A. 1972. "A new look at the mechanisms controlling sex differentiation in mammals." *Johns Hopkins Medical Journal*. Vol. 130: 38–53.

Koeske, Randi and Gary F. Koeske. 1975. "An attributional approach to moods and the menstrual cycle." *Journal of Personality and Social Psychology*. Vol. 31: 473–478.

Kopell, B. S., D. T. Lunde, R. B. Clayton and R. H. Moos. 1969. "The variations in some measures of arousal during the menstrual cycle." *Journal of Nervous and Mental Disorders*. Vol. 148: 180–187.

Kuriansky, Judith B. and Lawrence Sharpe. 1981. "Clinical and research implications of the evaluation of women's group therapy for anorgasmia: a review." *Journal of Sex and Marital Therapy*. Vol. 7: 268–277.

Kuriansky, Judith B., Lawrence Sharpe and Dagmar O'Connor. 1982. "The treatment of anorgasmia: long-term effectiveness of a short-term behavioral group therapy." *Journal of Sex and Marital Therapy*. Vol. 8: 29–43.

Lansdell, H. 1962. "A sex difference in effect of temporal-lobe neurosurgery on design preference." *Nature*. Vol. 194: 852–854.

Larned, D. 1974. "The Greening of the Womb." *New Times*. Vol. 2: 35–39.

Laros, R. K. 1975. "Female sterilization: A comparison of methods." *Obstetrics and Gynecology*. Vol. 46: 215–220.

Lembeke, A. 1956. "Medical Auditing by Scientific Methods: Illustrated by Major Pelvic Surgery." *Journal of the American Medical Association.* Vol. 162 (October): 646–655.

Lennane, Jean K., and John R. Lennane. 1973. "Alleged psychogenic disorders in women: A possible manifestation of sexual prejudice." *New England Journal of Medicine.* Vol. 288: 288–292.

Luttge, W. G. 1971. "The role of gonadal hormones in the sexual behavior of the rhesus monkey and human: A literature survey." *Archives of Sexual Behavior.* Vol. 1: 61.

Lyon, J. L. and J. W. Gardner. 1977. "The rising frequency of hysterectomy: Its effect on uterine cancer rates." *American Journal of Epidemiology.* Vol. 105: 439–443.

McCarthy, Eugene G. and Geraldine W. Widmar. 1974. "Effects of Screening by Consultants on Recommended Elective Surgical Procedures." *New England Journal of Medicine.* Vol. 291 (December): 1331–35.

McCarthy, E. G., and J. L. Finkel. 1980. "Second consultant opinion for elective gynecologic surgery." *Obstetrics and Gynecology.* Vol. 56: 403–410.

Marrett, L. D. 1980. "Estimates of the true population at risk of uterine disease and an application to incidence data of the uterine corpus in Connecticut." *American Journal of Epidemiology.* Vol. 111: 373–378.

Masson, Jeffrey M. 1984. "Freud and the Seduction Theory." *The Atlantic Monthly.* (February): 33–60.

Michael, Richard P., R. W. Bonsall and Patricia Warner. 1974. "Human vaginal secretions: Volatile fatty acid content." *Science.* Vol. 186 (December 24): 1217–1219.

Michael, R. P., E. B. Keverne and R. W. Bonsall. 1971. "Pheromones: Isolation of a male sex attractant from a female primate." *Science.* Vol. 172: 964–966.

Miller, N. F. 1946. "Hysterectomy: Therapeutic necessity or surgical racket?" *American Journal of Obstetrics and Gynecology.* Vol. 51: 804–810.

Parrott, M. H. 1972. "Elective hysterectomy." *American Journal of Obstetrics and Gynecology.* Vol. 113: 531–536.

Perry, B. W. 1976. "Time trends in hysterectomy 1970–1975." *PAS Reporter.* Vol. 14: 1–4.

Raglianti, P. 1980. "Hysterectomy and depression: a clinical study." *Bollettino di Psicologia Applicata.* (July-December): 205–211.

Reubens, Jacqueline R. 1982. "The physiology of normal sexual response in females." *Journal of Psychoactive Drugs.* (January-June): 45–46.

Reynolds, Evelyn. 1969. "Variations of mood and recall in the menstrual cycle." *Journal of Psychosomatic Research.* Vol. 13: 163–166.

Robinson, D. S., J. M. Davis, A. Nies, C. L. Ravaris and D. Sylvester. 1971. "Relation of sex and aging in monoamine oxidase activity of human brain, plasma and platelets." *Archives of General Psychiatry*. Vol. 24: 536–539.

Rochat, R. 1976. "Regional variation in sterility, United States." *Advances in Planned Parenthood*. Vol. 9: 1–11.

Rosenberg, L., C. H. Hennekens and B. Rosner. 1981. "Early menopause and the risk of myocardial infarction." *American Journal of Obstetrics and Gynecology*. Vol. 139: 47–51.

Roubicek, J., R. Tachezy and M. Matousek. 1968. "Electrical activity of the brain during the menstrual cycle." *Ceskoslovenska Psychiatrie*. Vol. 64: 90–94.

Roughan, Penelope A. and Lisbeth Kunst. 1981. "Do pelvic floor exercises really improve orgasmic potential?" *Journal of Sex and Marital Therapy*. Vol. 7: 223–229.

Shader, Richard I., Alberto Di Mascio and Jerold Harmatz. 1968. "Characterological anxiety levels and premenstrual libido changes." *Psychosomatics*. Vol. 9 (July-August): 197–198.

Sheldrake, Peter and Margaret Cormack. 1974. "Dream recall and the menstrual cycle." *Journal of Psychosomatic Research*. Vol. 18: 347–350.

Shepard, M. K. 1974. "Female contraceptive sterilization." *Obstetric Gynecological Survey*. Vol. 29: 739–787.

Skultans, Vieda. 1970. "The symbolic significance of menstruation and the menopause." *Man*. Vol. 5: 639–651.

Sommer, Barbara. 1973. "The effect of menstruation on cognitive and perceptual-motor behaviour: a review." *Psychosomatic Medicine*. Vol. 35: 515–534.

Subramaniam, Deepa, S. K. Subramaniam, S. X. Charles and Verghese Abraham. 1982. "Psychiatric aspects of hysterectomy." *Indian Journal of Psychiatry*. Vol. 24 (January): 75–79.

Thomas, W. L. 1953. "Prevenception insurance: Panhysterectomy versus tubectomy." *Southern Medical Journal*. Vol. 46: 787–791.

Walker, A. M. and H. Jick. 1979. "Temporal and regional variation in hysterectomy rates in the United States: 1970–1975." *American Journal of Epidemiology*. Vol. 110: 41–46.

Wennberg, J. E., J. P. Bunker and B. Barnes. 1980. "The need for assessing the outcome of common medical practices." *Annual Revue of Public Health*. Vol. 1: 277–295.

West, Joanne. 1983. "Estrogens: Yours, Theirs and the Horse's." *Hers Newsletter*. (July): 2–4.

Whitelaw, C. A. 1979. "Ten-year survey of 485 sterilizations: Part I. Sterilization or hysterectomy?" *British Medical Journal*. Vol. 1: 32–33.

Wineman, E. W. 1971. "Autonomic balance changes during the human menstrual cycle." *Psychophysiology*. Vol. 8: 1–6.

Wright, R. C. 1969. "Hysterectomy: past, present and future." *Obstetrics and Gynecology*. Vol. 33: 560–563.

Yalom, I. D., R. Green and N. Fisk. 1973. "Prenatal exposure to female hormones: effect on psychosexual development in boys." *Archives of General Psychiatry*. Vol. 28: 554–561.

Young, W. C. 1965. "The organization of sexual behavior by hormonal action during the prenatal and larval periods in vertebrates." *Sex and Behavior*. 000: 89–107.

Zimmerman, Ellen and Mary Brown Parlee. 1973. "Behavioural changes associated with the menstrual cycle: an experimental investigation." *Journal of Applied Social Psychology*. Vol. 3: 335–344.

Zwerner, Janna. 1982. "Yes, we have troubles but nobody's listening: sexual issues of women with spinal cord injury." *Sexuality and Disability*. Vol. 5 (Fall): 158–171.

Reports

American College of Obstetricians and Gynecologists. 1977. *Executive Board Statement of Policy*. Washington, D.C.

———. 1985. *Public Information*. Washington, D.C.

Atlanta Centers for Disease Control. 1980. *Surgical Sterilization Surveillance: Hysterectomy 1970–1975*. Atlanta, GA: U.S. Government Printing Office.

———. 1981. *Surgical Sterilization Surveillance: Hysterectomy 1976–1978*. Atlanta, GA: U.S. Government Printing Office.

Bishop, Dr. J. Michael. 1983. Speech to the American Association of Medical Colleges.

House Subcommittee on Oversight and Investigations of the Committee on Interstate and Foreign Commerce. 1976. *Cost and Quality of Health Care: Unnecessary Surgery*. Washington, D.C.: U.S. Government Printing Office.

Korenbrot, Carol, Ann B. Flood, Michael Higgins, Noralou Roos and John P. Bunker. 1981. *The Implications of Cost-Effectiveness Analysis of Medical Technology. Case Study #15: Elective Hysterectomy: Costs, Risks, and Benefits*. San Francisco: Division of Health Services Research, Stanford University.

Metropolitan Life Insurance Co. 1985. *Annual Report*. New York.

Torjman, Dr. Gilbert. 1983. A paper presented as the president of the World Association for Sexology, at the Sixth World Congress of Sexology. Washington, D.C.

U.S. Bureau of the Census. 1979. *Fertility of American Women: June 1978, Current Population Reports, Series P-20, No. 341*. Washington, D.C.: U.S. Government Printing Office.

U.S. Department of Health and Human Services. 1970. *Development of the Design of the NCHS Hospital Discharge Survey: Vital and Health Statistics, series 2, No. 39*. Rockville, MD: National Center for Health Statistics.

U.S. Department of Health and Human Services. 1967. *Eighth Revision International Classification of Disease. Adapted for Use in the United States.* Rockville, MD: National Center for Health Statistics.

————. 1983. *Fecundity and Infertility in the United States: 1965–82.* Hyattsville, MD: U.S. Government Printing Office.

————. 1984. *1983 Summary: National Hospital Discharge Survey.* National Center for Health Statistics. Hyattsville, MD: U.S. Government Printing Office.

————. 1983. *Vital and Health Statistics.* Hyattsville, MD: U.S. Government Printing Office.

Audio Visual

Public Concept Media. 1975. *Surgical Procedures: Impact on Sexuality.* Slide and audio cassette. Costa Mesa, CA.

Index

Medical indications for hysterectomy, 45–56
Medical schools, 77–78, 89, 145, 146, 180
Medicare, 46, 92
Medicine, history of, 142–158
Medroxyprogesterone acetate, 87
Melges, Frederick T., 76
Men, hysterectomy and, 135–140
Menopause, 8, 183–184
Menstruation, 5, 95–98, 100–107, 110, 115
Mentuhetep, Queen, 143
Microsurgery techniques, 33
Midwives, 143–144, 147, 148
Mississippi Appendectomy, 38
Mitchell, S. Weir, 154–156
Moontide, 107
Morris, N. M., 115
Mortality rates, 43
Myomectomy, 56, 168

National Center for Health Statistics (NCHS), 35–36, 40
New Our Bodies, Ourselves, The (Boston Women's Health Book Collective), 89, 170
Newton, Niles, 59
Nutrition, 170, 171

Omentum, 54
On Being a Woman (Gifford-Jones), 60, 61
On the Generation of Animals (Aristotle), 101–102
Oophorectomy, 10, 34, 36, 37, 39–40, 42–43, 49, 50, 56, 57, 59, 72–74, 79, 169, 172, 183
Operative complications, 44
Orgasm, 59, 61–63, 66, 67, 70, 84, 106, 121, 123–126, 130–133, 177, 179
Osteoporosis, 3–4, 172

Ovarian cancer, 39–40, 42, 54–55, 161
Ovarian cycle, 104
Ovarian hormones, 109, 111–115, 122–123
Ovid, 147
Oxytocin, 112

Pan hysterectomy, defined, 49
PAP examinations, 42
Paracelsus, 149
Pars intermedia, 112
Pars nervosa, 112
Partial mastectomy, 45
Peer review, 47
Pellet implantation, 172
Pelvic exenterations, 34
Pelvic Inflammatory Disease, 49, 53, 161
Penile implants, 86
Peptides, 118
Peritonitis, 72
Periurethral glands, 124
Physical fitness, 174–175
Pituitary gland, 112, 113
Plastic surgery, 33
Plautus, 147
Pliny, 97, 143, 147
Posthysterectomy syndrome, 4, 30, 35, 45, 81, 137, 139, 165, 172
    See also Sexual desire, loss of
Postoperative complications, 44
Premenstrual syndrome (PMS), 103, 105–106
Prodomal menopausal state, 56
Professional Standards Review Organizations (PSRO), 45–47
Progesterone, 87, 104, 105, 111, 115, 117–119
Progestins, 111
Prolactin, 112
Prolapsed uterus, 42, 45, 47, 49, 53, 164

About the Author

Naomi Miller Stokes, wife, mother, and grandmother, began as a magazine and newspaper writer and went on to own and run an advertising agency for twenty-five years. Since 1982 she has devoted her time to writing and lecturing. She lives in Portland, Oregon.